Atlas of Dynamic Laryngeal Pathology

Atlas of Dynamic Laryngeal Pathology

C. Richard Stasney, M.D., F.A.C.S.

Director, Texas Voice Center
Director, The Van Lawrence Voice Institute, Baylor College of Medicine
Clinical Associate Professor of Otolaryngology, Baylor College of Medicine
Adjunct Professor, Linguistics Deptartment, Rice University

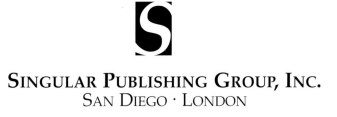

SINGULAR PUBLISHING GROUP, INC.
SAN DIEGO · LONDON

Singular Publishing Group, Inc.
401 West A Street, Suite 325
San Diego, California 92101-7904

19 Compton Terrace
London, N1 2UN, United Kingdom

© 1996 Singular Publishing Group, Inc.

Typeset in 11/13 Palatino by So Cal Graphics
Printed in Hong Kong by Paramount Printing Company

All rights, including that of translation, reserved. No part of this publication may be reproduced, stored in a retrieval system, or transmitted in any form or by any means, electronic, mechanical, recording, or otherwise, without the prior written permission of the publisher.

ISBN 1-56593-622-1

Contributors

J. David Garrett, Ph.D., C.C.C. SLP.
Voice Physiologist and Speech-Language Pathologist
Texas Voice Center and the Van Lawrence Voice Institute at Baylor
Assistant Professor, Otolaryngology Head and
Neck Surgery,
Baylor College of Medicine
Adjunct Professor, Linguistics Department, Rice University
Dr. Garrett's contributions to the functional analysis of the effect of the pathology on the voice
using the videostroboscopy and
Kay Multi-Dimensional Voice Program (MDVP) are under the
Pathophysiology sections.

Sharon L. Radionoff, Ph.D.
Singing Voice Specialist and Voice Technologist,
Texas Voice Center
Lecturer, Shepherd School of Music, Rice University

Margarita Rodriguez, B.S.
Medical Clinic Coordinator, Videostroboscopy Technician and Archivist,
Texas Voice Center

dedicated to the memory of three giants
in the field of Laryngology
Friedrich S. Brodnitz, M.D.
Wilbur James Gould, M.D.
Van Lawrence, M.D.
on whose shoulders we stand.

Contents

Preface	xi
Introduction to Laryngeal Pathophysiology	1
I. **Normal Larynx**	5
II. **Anatomic Variations of the Larynx**	11
III. **Functional Abnormalities of the Larynx**	12
IV. **Benign Lesions**	23
A. Prenodules	23
B. Nodules	24
C. Polyps	31
D. Cysts and Laryngoceles	37
E. Edema	42
F. Ulcers and Granulomas	46
G. Inflammation	54
H. Vascular Pathologies	66
V. **Vocal Fold Concavity**	68
VI. **Traumatic Pathology**	71
VII. **Scarring of the Larynx**	74
A. Webs	74
B. Stenosis	79
C. Adynamic Vocal Fold Segment	83
D. Vocal Fold Notching	84
VIII. **Tumors**	86
A. Benign	86
B. Premalignant (Hyperkeratosis and Leukoplakia)	91
C. Malignant	94
D. Invasive Carcinoma	95

IX. Neurologic Disorders — 101
- A. Nerve Paresis and Paralysis — 101
- B. Spasmodic Dysphonia — 105
- C. Miscellaneous Neurological Disorders — 107

X. Hormonal Imbalances — 108

XI. Pediatric Laryngeal Disorders — 110
- A. Nodules — 111
- B. Polyps — 114
- C. Cysts — 115

Epilogue — 116
References — 117

Preface

The raison d'être for this interactive video-text is to assist the reader (viewer) in developing diagnostic skills for evaluating laryngeal pathology by demonstrating, through static and "slow motion video images," the larynx in health and in certain disease states.

At the onset, it must be made clear that many of the diagnoses included in this atlas are not clearly delineated in any single text printed to date. For example, there is a controversy about the distinction between nodules and polyps and their respective definitions. This treatise attempts to differentiate lesions from both a pathophysiological and a histological perspective.

In addition, in several cases, results from Kay Elemetrics Multi-Dimensional Voice Program will be depicted. While it is understood that each Multi-Dimensional Diagram (MDD) is specific to the case being shown, until we have much more data, any attempt to infer what is a "typical" pattern for that particular condition awaits. Also, several examples may have no effect on the voice (e.g., normal variants of corniculate cartilages, subglottic Wegener's, etc.) and, therefore, present with no abnormalities in voice analysis. The staff at the Texas Voice Center feel it is important to introduce this new technology and to show the studies done on many of the cases shown.

The equipment used for Computer Speech Lab analysis of the voice is the Kay Model 4300B CSL. The predominant videolaryngostroboscopy equipment is the Kay Model RLS 9100 Video Strobe with a 70° Kay rigid telescope. A few of the older cases were videostrobed using the Brüel and Kjaer Rhino-Larynx Stroboscope Type 4914 with a Nagashima 90° rigid telescope model SFT-I. Occasionally, the flexible Olympus ENF type P3 laryngocope is used.

Introduction to Laryngeal Pathophysiology

Over the last several decades the development of new technologies and new techniques has revolutionized the field of voice care. This is especially true when one is attempting to determine the functional effects of the pathology on the voice. Improvements in the videostroboscopy equipment have greatly enhanced the ability to accurately assess how a particular pathology is affecting the ability of the vocal folds to vibrate in a normal way. Similarly, acoustic analyses of the voice, which were previously used primarily as a research tool, are now becoming a valuable tool for clinicians in the field.

It is our belief that the increased speed with which acoustic analyses can be performed, combined with a greater understanding of how to interpret the acoustic parameters, ultimately will result in a powerful tool for clinicians to use in the field. Significant efforts by our voice team and others are underway to more fully understand how the different acoustic parameters relate to the vocal fold vibrations and how the parameters change in response to laryngeal pathologies. Because knowledge of how to fully interpret acoustic parameters is incomplete, the analogy of the glass being half empty or half full may be appropriate. One could easily argue that the incomplete nature of our understanding of the acoustic parameters serves as a detriment to the use of these parameters as a clinical tool. If, on the other hand, the glass is viewed as half full, the use of acoustic analysis is already capable of providing important information about how the vocal folds are vibrating, and consistent use of acoustic parameters will increase the depth of knowledge for the future.

A number of programs that perform sophisticated analyses of the voice are currently available. The analyses presented in this text were performed using the Kay Elemetrics MDVP (Multi-Dimensional Voice Program) Model 4305. One of the benefits of this program is the method used to represent the acoustic parameters. A polar diagram is used in which each parameter is graphed as a line extending from a central point. Each diagram represents sustained phonation of the /ɑ/ vowel. The point where the green circle intersects each line represents the normal threshold for each parameter. If the value of the parameter is greater than the normal threshold, the trace extends outside of the circle and is shown in red. The advantage of this form of representation, which will be referred to as the "MDD" or Multi-Dimensional Diagram, is that clinicians can quickly determine which values are excessive. Another advantage is that it enhances the clinicians' ability to use all of the available information and begin to recognize different "patterns." Below is the list of the parameters and the explanations of the parameters provided by Kay Elemetrics. Following this list is a more general explanation of how to view the MDD for those who have less experience with acoustic parameters.

Short-term and Long-term Frequency Perturbation Measurements

Jita—*Absolute Jitter* gives an evaluation of the period-to-period variability of the pitch period within the analyzed voice sample.

Jitt—*Jitter Percent* gives an evaluation of the variability of the pitch period within the analyzed voice sample. It represents the relative period-to-period (very short-term) variability.

RAP—*Relative Average Perturbation* gives an evaluation of the variability of the pitch period within the analyzed voice sample at a smoothing factor of 3 periods.

PPQ—*Pitch Period Perturbation Quotient* gives an evaluation of the variability of the pitch period within the analyzed voice sample at a smoothing factor of 5 periods.

sPPQ—*Smoothed Pitch Period Perturbation Quotient* gives an evaluation of the short-term or long-term variability of the pitch period within the analyzed voice sample. The smoothing factor was set at 55 periods.

vFo—*Fundamental Frequency Variation* represents the relative standard deviation of the period-to-period calculated fundamental frequency. It reflects the very long-term variations of F_0 for all the analyzed sample.

Short-term and Long-term Amplitude Perturbation Measurements

ShdB—*Shimmer in dB* gives an evaluation of the period-to-period variability of the peak-to-peak amplitude within the analyzed voice sample.

Shim—*Shimmer Percent* gives an evaluation of the variability of the peak-to-peak amplitude within the analyzed voice sample. It represents the relative period-to-period (very short-term) variability of the peak-to-peak amplitude.

APQ—*Amplitude Perturbation Quotient* gives an evaluation of the variability of the peak-to-peak amplitude within the analyzed voice sample at smoothing factor of 11 periods.

sAPQ—*Smoothed Amplitude Perturbation Quotient* gives an evaluation of the short-term or long-term variability of the peak-to-peak amplitude within the analyzed voice sample. The smoothing factor was set at 55 periods but can be set by the user.

vAm—*Peak Amplitude Variation* represents the relative standard deviation of the period-to-period calculated peak-to-peak amplitude. It reflects the very long-term amplitude variations within the analyzed voice sample.

Voice Break Related Measurements

DVB—*Degree of Voice Breaks* shows in percent the ratio of the total length of areas representing voice breaks to the time of the complete voice sample.

Sub-Harmonic Components Related Measurements

DSH—*Degree of Sub-Harmonics* is an estimated relative evaluation of sub-harmonic to F_0 components in the voice sample.

Voice Irregularity Related Measurements

DUV—*Degree of Voiceless* is an estimated relative evaluation of non-harmonic areas (where F_0 cannot be detected) in the voice sample.

Noise Related Measurements

NHR—*Noise-to-Harmonic Ratio* is an average ratio of energy of the inharmonic components in the range of 1500–4500 Hz to the harmonic components energy in the range of 70–4500 Hz. It is a general evaluation of the noise presence in the analyzed signal (such as amplitude and frequency variations, turbulence noise, subharmonic components and/or voice breaks).

VTI—*Voice Turbulence Index* is an average ratio of the spectral inharmonic high frequency energy in the range 2800–5800 Hz to the spectral harmonic energy in the range 70–4500 Hz in the areas of the signal where the influence of the frequency and amplitude variations, voice breaks and subharmonic components are minimal. VTI measures the relative energy level of high frequency noise. It mostly correlates with turbulence.

SPI—*Soft Phonation Index* This parameter is not actually a measurement of noise, but rather the harmonic structure of the spectrum. It is an average ratio of the lower frequency harmonic energy (70–1600 Hz) to the higher frequency (1600–4500 Hz) harmonic energy. Increased value of SPI may be an indication of incomplete or loosely adducted folds during phonation.

Tremor Measurements

FTRI—F_0 *Tremor Intensity Index* shows in percent the ratio of the frequency magnitude of the most intensive low frequency modulating component (F_0 tremor) to the total frequency magnitude of the analyzed voice signal.

ATRI—*Amplitude Tremor Intensity Index* shows in percent the ratio of the amplitude of the most intensive low frequency amplitude modulating component (amplitude tremor) to the total amplitude of the analyzed voice signal.

Explanation of the Parameters

Please note that these descriptions are highly simplified to provide a basic understanding of how the parameters relate to the vocal folds. Cases 1 and 2 may be used as a reference for normal phonation of an /ɑ/ vowel.

When looking at the MDD, the values from the 12 o'clock position moving clockwise to the 3 o'clock position refer to the frequency perturbation. During the production of a sustained vowel, normal vocal folds should open and close at the same rate from cycle to cycle. That is, it should take the same amount of time for one cycle to occur as the next. These parameters will increase if the rate of the vibrations change from cycle to cycle. In general, as you go from the 12 to the 3 o'clock position, the first few parameters (Jita, Jitt, RAP, PPQ) look for very short-term cycle-to-cycle changes. The remaining parameters (sPPQ and vFo) look at variations in the cycle-to-cycle rate that are more long term in nature.

The values that move from the 3 to the 6 o'clock positions are organized similarly, except that these parameters are testing the amplitude perturbation. During the production of a sustained vowel, normal vocal folds should open to the same width from cycle to cycle. These parameters will increase if the width of the opening changes from cycle to cycle. The short-term measures are the ShdB, Shim, and APQ; the sAPQ and vAm represent long-term variations in the amplitude.

Continuing clockwise around the circle, the next two parameters (NHR and VTI) are noise-related measurements. Extra noise in the signal can come from a number of sources. These include amplitude and frequency variations and turbulence noise from excessive air flow through the glottis. The measure of SPI is also related to the amount of high frequency energy and may relate to consistent air leakage, but the meaning of this parameter is unknown at this time.

The next two parameters (FTRI and ATRI) determine if there is low frequency modulation of the frequency (pitch) or amplitude (loudness) of the signal. These values increase if there is a regularity to the changes such as occurs when tremor or vibrato is present.

The remainder of the values (DVB, DSH, DUV) relate to times where there are voice breaks in the signal or when subharmonics are detected in the signal.

I. NORMAL LARYNX

Case 1: Normal adult male

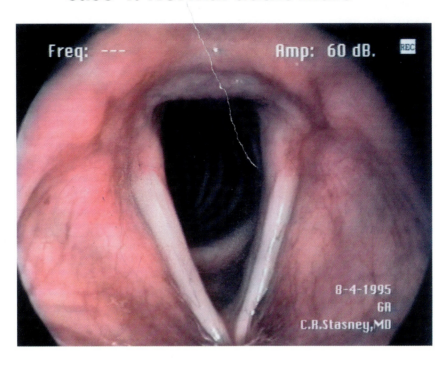

The first case is a 38-year-old male voice scientist with a normal voice and normal videostroboscopic examination of the larynx. Appreciation of the subtleties of videostroboscopy and its value in assessing laryngeal function necessitates that the viewer has a certain knowledge of the technology involved. There follows a brief overview of videostroboscopy to facilitate this understanding.

The human retina can absorb approximately five images per second. Obviously, at the "middle C" rate in the proximity of 262 Hertz (262 vocal fold cycles per second), the action is much too fast to be visualized by the human eye. Videostroboscopy takes advantage of the retina's physiology by causing light bursts at different phases of the vibratory cycle, thereby giving the effect of "slow-motion." This ability to visualize the vocal folds in quasi slow-motion allows us to make the following qualitative and quantitative evaluations of glottic performance (the normal physiologic response is italicized):

1. **Vocal fold edge:** varies from *smooth and straight* to rough and irregular (primarily refers to the phonating margin)
2. **Glottic closure:** *complete*, anterior chink, irregular closure, bowing, posterior chink, hour glass, or incomplete (as in "railroad track" vocal folds)
3. **Phase closure:** varies from open phase predominates (whisper) to *normal* to closed phase predominates (hyperadduction)
4. **Vertical level of vocal folds:** *equal*, right lower, left lower
5. **Amplitude:** *normal* to diminished to absent (this refers to maximum excursion of the vocal folds during phonation)
6. **Mucosal wave:** *normal* to absent (normal means that the wave travels approximately 50% across the upper fold when at the fundamental frequency)
7. **Phase symmetry:** *regular* to mostly irregular (ideally, the vocal folds will mirror image each other and move symmetrically)
8. **Periodicity:** *regular* to always irregular (there should be regular, rhythmic, metronome type oscillation of the folds)
9. **Ventricular folds:** *normal* to full compression (dysphonia plica ventricularis); the ventricular folds (or false cords) should be

relatively immobile and apart during phonation

10. **Arytenoids:** *normal* to poor movement (the arytenoids should move symmetrically, both during adduction and abduction)
11. **Hyperfunction:** *not present* to always present (watch particularly the supraglottic structures and for anterior-posterior as well as lateral-medial compression of the larynx)

Medical diagnoses are based primarily on these videostroboscopic findings and the appearance of the causative lesions. Rigid examination gives the most information vis-à-vis medical diagnoses. Additional findings from flexible videolaryngoscopy allow more functional information of particular benefit to speech-language pathologists and singing voice specialists.

The various phases of closure will be seen in this composite digitized video image (Fig a). When viewing the video example, the cycling of normal vocal folds is apparent in the case of this 38-year-old male voice scientist with a fundamental frequency of 105 hertz. One notes the phase symmetry (mirror image movement of the folds), the regular repetition of the cycles (periodicity), the traveling mucosal wave (approximately one half the superior fold surface near the optimal fundamental frequency), the lack of movement of the false folds, the normal motion of the arytenoids, and the smooth edges of the vocal folds. There is no apparent hyperfunction and the entire fold is easily visualized without the appearance of constriction (either in an anterior-posterior dimension or from the sides).

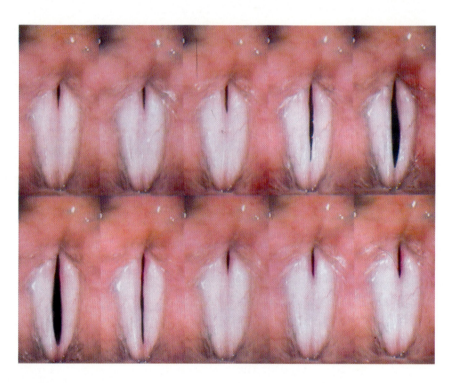

Fig a

Pathophysiology

Cases 1 and 2 are provided to familiarize the viewer with normal phonation and provide a baseline for viewing the various pathologies. Perceptually, the clarity of the vocal quality is readily apparent. The stroboscopy demonstrates regular periodic vocal fold vibrations. The rate at which the folds vibrate remains stable, which is consistent with the minimal amount of pitch perturbation seen on the MDD. The width that the folds open during each cycle is normal and stable from cycle to cycle, which is consistent with the minimal amount of amplitude perturbation seen on the MDD. The edges of the vocal folds during phonation demonstrate normal mucosal waves. Mucosal wave analysis provides valuable information for the clinician because an abnormal mucosal wave is often the first sign of a vocal fold problem. By comparing the mucosal waves of both folds simultaneously, it can be seen that they are moving symmetrically, thereby demonstrating a high phase symmetry. During the closed phase of the cycle, the vocal folds close along the entire extent of the folds except for a minor gap between the arytenoids. The gap is common in normals and tends to occur more often in females than in males. During the sample the frequency (perceived as pitch) is increased. Notice how the length of the folds is increased and the vibrating edges become thinner and more taut.

The perceptual quality of the voice and the stroboscopy findings are consistent with the MDD pattern (see Introduction to Laryngeal Physiology section). The parameters of the MDD are represented by a polar diagram in which each parameter is graphed as a line extending out from a central point. The point where the green circle intersects each line represents the normal threshold for each parameter. Notice how all of the values are within the normal threshold.

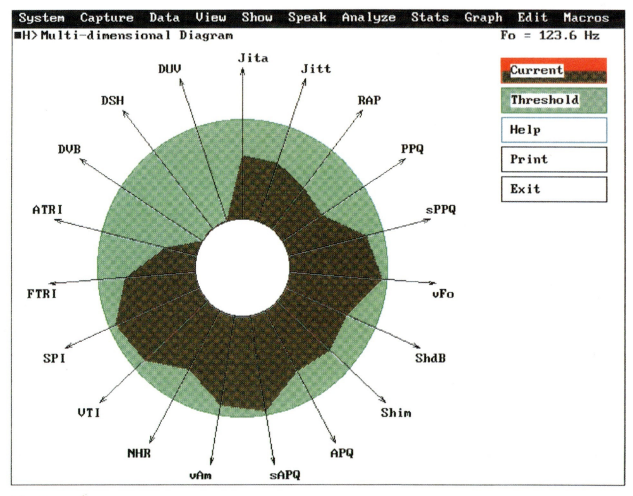

Fig 1

Case 2: Normal adult female

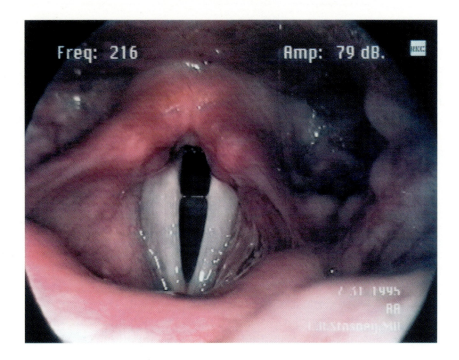

Note the pearly white vocal folds in this 34-year-old female classical singer (mezzo-soprano). The phonating margins of the vocal folds are straight (although a small amount of irregularity is within normal limits). The mucosal waves in the rigid examination travel at least 50% of the width of the fold and are quite symmetric. Note also that the amplitude of the arytenoid movement is normal and the arytenoids do not close in a "pressed fashion," preserving a "Gothic Arch" posteriorly and superiorly (on the video screen). Dr. Van Lawrence was fond of this description for the appearance of the posterior commissure when the larynx is performing at optimal level.

Pathophysiology

Figure 2a is an example of normal spoken phonation of the /ɑ/ vowel. Note that all of the parameters fall within the threshold values. Figure 2b is an example of normal sung phonation of the /ɑ/ vowel with vibrato. There are six parameters that fall outside of the normal threshold limits. Although these parameters are greater than the normal threshold, they do not indicate any abnormal voicing as these parameters reflect long-term variation in the pitch and amplitude that is characteristic of the production of vibrato.

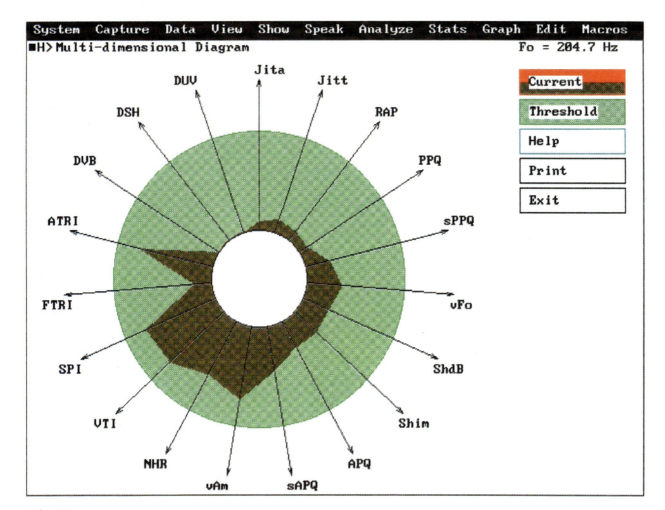

Fig 2A

Case 2 *(continued)*

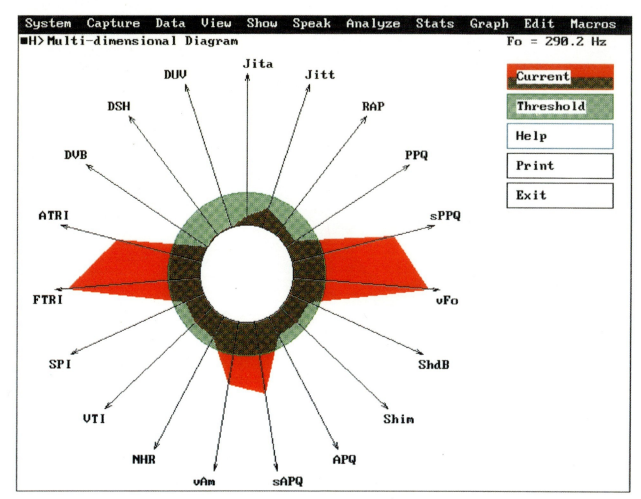

Fig 2B

II. ANATOMIC VARIATIONS OF THE LARYNX

Case 3: Corniculate/arytenoid

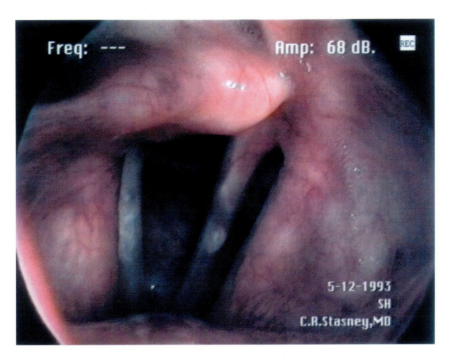

This case is of a 38-year-old businessman with a normal voice. Note the irregularities in symmetry of the corniculate cartilages in this patient. If the patient presented with dysphonia, one might incorrectly infer that he suffers from a dislocated arytenoid/corniculate complex. Obviously, there is a wide variation in the human larynx and the possibility of dislocations and abnormalities should be carefully substantiated by further studies.

III. FUNCTIONAL ABNORMALITIES OF THE LARYNX

Case 4: Hypofunction

Note, in this case of a 10-year-old female student, that the folds are sluggish and do not approximate quickly and firmly. There is a persistent 2–3 mm gap producing a very breathy and weak voice even with increasing pitch and amplitude. The patient responded to speech therapy, and later studies demonstrated normal laryngeal function with normal fold contact and a much stronger voice.

Pathophysiology

The arytenoids, in the posterior region of the vocal folds, never approximate completely during voicing. This results in a posterior gap that allows air to consistently escape, thereby producing a breathy sounding voice. The additional air escaping wastes air which shortens the maximum phonation times. The posterior gap extends from one-third the length of the folds and frequently increases to extend the length of the folds, preventing any vocal fold vibrations. The best vibrations occur at the initiation of each phonation when the gap is the smallest and the breath support is the best. Following this initial period, the muscular forces reduce at a steady rate. Therefore, the longer the voicing sample, the less vibrations and more breathy the voicing becomes.

Case 5: Hyperfunction

This example is given by a 38-year-old male voice scientist who is feigning hyperfunction. Note that there is quick, firm closure of the cords and lateral compression of the false vocal folds. The supraglottic structures should remain relatively static during phonation and the full width and length of the true folds visible when phonating at the patient's fundamental frequency. In its most severe degree, hyperfunction results in dysphonia plica ventricularis, or phonation with the false vocal folds. This case demonstrates predominately lateral compression, whereas the next case predominately demonstrates anterior-posterior compression when hyperfunction is displayed.

Pathophysiology

Hyperfunction refers to excessive muscular tension. In the beginning of this sample, there is both anterior-posterior constriction and medial-lateral constriction. The anterior-posterior constriction typically is characterized by the arytenoids being pulled too far anteriorly. Often, a hump is seen at the base of the epiglottis near the anterior commissure. The medial-lateral constriction typically is characterized by increased medialization of the ventricular (false) folds which obscures the width of the true folds. In this sample, when the physician asks for less hyperfunction, the anterior-posterior constriction is reduced and almost eliminated (the arytenoids move posteriorly) leaving, primarily, the anterior-posterior constriction.

Case 6: Hyperfunction

In this case (a 34-year-old female classical singer) note that the false folds are relatively static; however, the true folds are compressed in the anterior-posterior dimension and they meet along each edge with a ferocity. The ensuing sound is pressed and stressed. One can see how this behavior is conducive to damage along the phonating margins.

Pathophysiology

This case of severe hyperfunction demonstrates both anterior-posterior and medial-lateral constriction (see case 5), although the former predominates. The effects of the excessive tension on the vocal fold vibrations are very apparent. The vocal folds are so severely compressed that the majority of the vocal fold cycle is taken up by the closed phase. This results in the strained/strangled sound of the voice. In the second portion of the sample, the hyperfunction is reduced, demonstrating the way in which the open phase increases, resulting in a less strained/strangled voice.

Case 7: Hyperfunction

In this case, that of a 40-year-old female speech-language pathologist, a general constriction of the supraglottic structures is seen with lateral and anterior-posterior compression. One can hear the effects of this hyperfunction on the speaking voice and see the etiology via the flexible laryngoscope.

Pathophysiology

Both anterior-posterior and medial-lateral constriction are readily seen in this sample. Medial-lateral constriction is characterized by the medialization of the ventricular folds and occurs primarily at, or just prior to, the initial sound of words.

Case 8: Hyperfunction

During this song performed by a 34-year-old female classical singer, one hears the constricted sound replete with tension. These functional abnormalities are evident during the flexible laryngoscopy. Gone is the "Gothic Arch" Dr. Van Lawrence used to describe the shape of the aryepiglottic folds combined with the arytenoids and the posterior commissure when the patient is phonating without stress at the patient's optimal fundamental frequency.

Case 9: Hyperfunction—posterior chink

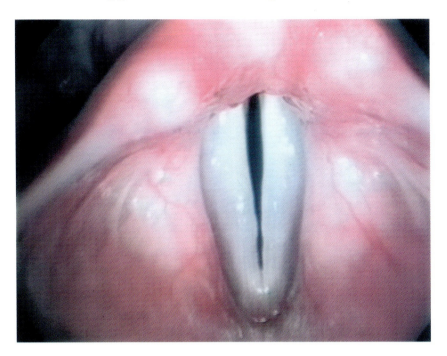

This 25-year-old female classical singer demonstrates typical hyperfunction. She has a persistent posterior chink between the vocal processes of the arytenoids. One hypothesis for this gap is that it represents a continuous contraction of the posterior cricoarytenoid muscle which never relaxes completely and, therefore, causes a small posterior aperture. It is far more common in females and is associated with prenodules and nodules. One other hypothesis for this phenomenon is that there is an overcontraction of the interarytenoid muscle. This results in abduction of the vocal processes of the arytenoids as the arytenoids overclose.

Pathophysiology

The arytenoids fail to approximate at any time, even at the higher pitches. The gap results in excess air escaping and the voice being breathy. Another important aspect of this vocal fold configuration is that all of the acoustic (sound) energy is being produced by the anterior half of the vocal folds, placing increased demands on this area.

Case 10: Dysphonia plica ventricularis

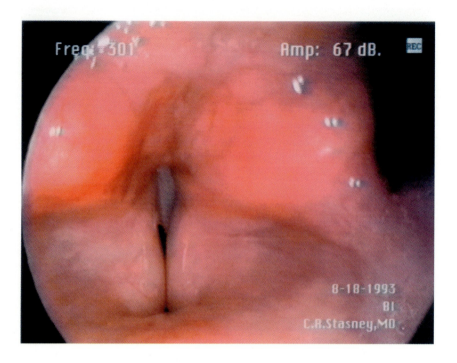

This case demonstrates an extreme form of hyperfunction in an 88-year-old female. It is an exaggerated form of hyperfunction with closure of the false vocal folds (and phonation effected by them). Many times, as in this case, the patient is elderly and has presbylaryngis with an incomplete closure of the true folds. In these instances, dysphonia plica ventricularis may be an attempt to achieve oscillations by surface contact of other laryngeal structures.

Pathophysiology

This extreme form of hyperfunction occurs when the medial tension is so severe that the ventricular (false) folds approximate and begin to vibrate. When the ventricular folds vibrate, it is usually at a very low frequency due to the mass and location of these structures. The sound produced by two pair of folds vibrating simultaneously at different pitches is often referred to as diplophonia. During speech, the tension increases and the ventricular vibrations tend to become more prominent at the same time that the pitch drops (e.g., at the ends of words, phrases, or sentences). The medial compression of the ventricular folds often becomes so severe that it results in complete glottic closure. Often, patients report that the voice "quits" or "gives out."

Case 11: Functional aphonia

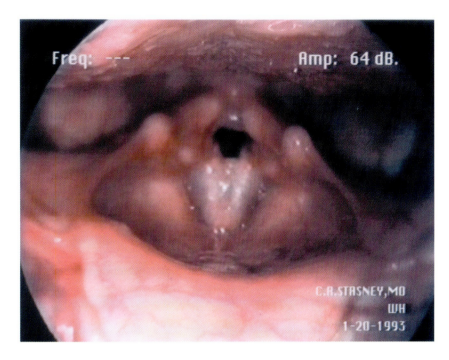

In this case, a 41-year-old female manual laborer was exposed to an explosion in a petrochemical plant 2 years prior and has not phonated since. The appearance of the larynx is much as it would be for a "stage whisper" with a keyhole gap between the arytenoids. Coughing and clearing the throat, the patient could close the interarytenoid gap. Many times, functional (or hysterical) aphonia is a form of conversion reaction and psychiatric help is very important once organic etiologies have been excluded. One senior laryngologist, a friend of the author, would tell the patient that his or her larynx was "dislocated." He would then proceed to manipulate the larynx in the neck and then say to the patient: "Now the dislocation has been reduced and you can talk." Astonishingly, he cured about 50% of the cases of hysterical aphonia he treated using this technique.

Pathophysiology

The tips of the vocal processes of the arytenoids are tightly compressed medially. The posterior portion of the arytenoids remain open, resulting in a triangular posterior chink. The air rushing through the chink results in turbulence of the air, producing the whisper-like sound. No vocal fold vibrations are present in this sample.

Case 12: Functional aphonia

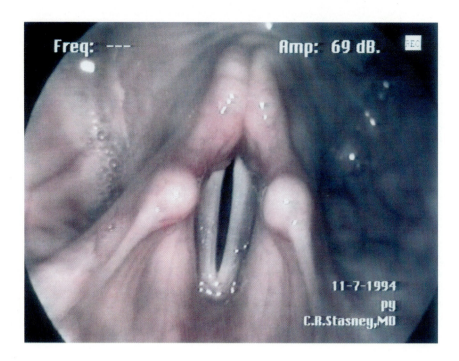

This patient (a 31-year-old female registered nurse) suffered a complete loss of speech following an emotional trauma several months prior. Conversion reactions such as this are sometimes best treated by psychiatric help; however, with insight gleaned from the videostroboscopy and speech therapy, her voice was restored during the first office visit. Note the way in which the folds approximate when the patient coughs, a sign that the lack of closure is functional.

Pathophysiology

Notice the way in which the posterior region of the arytenoid cartilages are brought together and the vocal processes remain open. The most likely explanation for this vocal fold configuration is muscular activity occurring in the abductor muscles (posterior cricoarytenoid) with little activity from the adductors (lateral cricoarytenoid and thyroarytenoid muscles). The only adductor muscles contracting are the interarytenoids which bring the posterior region of the arytenoids together. The failure to bring the vocal processes together combined with little tension from within the vocal folds results in the lack of approximation of the folds, preventing any vibration. The tight production of the cough is evidence that the adductor muscles have sufficient strength and control to phonate when used properly.

The acoustic analysis (Fig 12, a) confirms what is seen with the stroboscopy. Approximately half of the sample is non-voiced and the signal is made up primarily of spectral inharmonic high-frequency energy due to the air rushing through the open glottis. This can be seen by the lack of frequency and amplitude tracking and the extremely high value of voice turbulence index on the MDD (Fig 12, b). The vocal folds vibrate intermittently, but the vibrations are rarely periodic as seen by the extremely high jitter and shimmer values on the MDD. This is due to the fact that the vocal folds are vibrating independently because they fail to approximate at the midline.

Case 12 *(continued)*

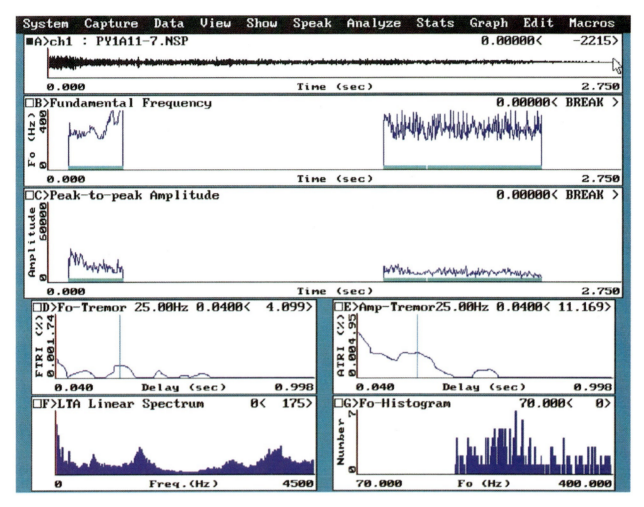

Fig 12B

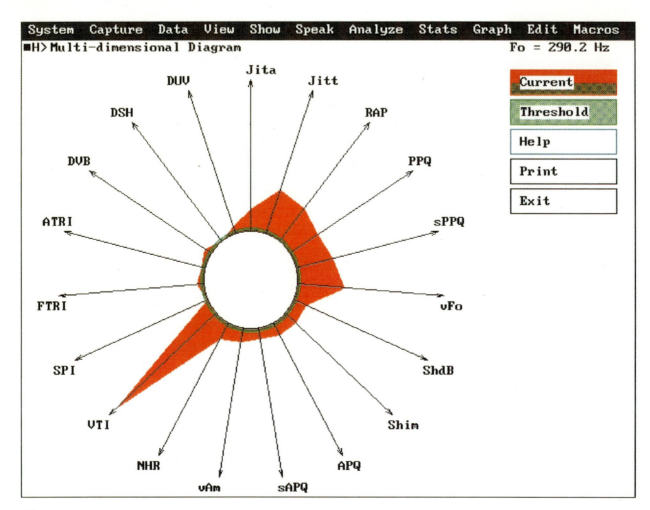

Fig 12A

IV. BENIGN LESIONS

A. Prenodules

Case 13: Prenodules

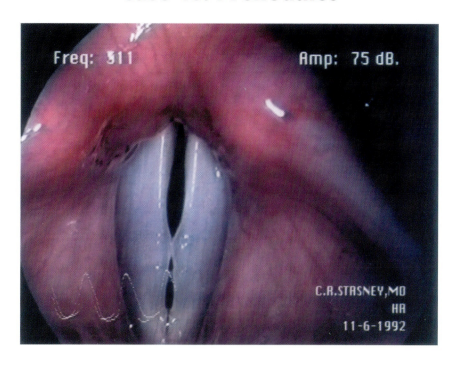

In the case of this 29-year-old female classical singer, one sees swelling at the junction of the anterior and middle thirds of the vocal folds. These lesions are often referred to as "soft nodules." Lesions like this can be physiological and last for approximately 24 hours following a particularly difficult Verdi or Puccini role. In this particular case, the prenodules resulted from errors in speaking and singing technique and abated when these deficiencies were corrected. The electroglottography demonstrated in the lower left quadrant of the screen theoretically reflects closure of the vocal folds, but there are so many variables in this test (skin conductivity, position of electrodes, amount of subcutaneous tissue, etc.) that this author has abandoned routine electroglottography.

An important addendum to this treatise is to admonish the reader to be very careful in using the term "vocal nodules." This has the emotional impact of telling a singer that he or she has cancer. Most laryngologists use euphemisms such as "prenodular swelling," "physiological swelling," "singer's callouses," and so on.

Pathophysiology

These swellings are very pliable, allowing fairly regular mucosal waves. The most significant problem is that all of the acoustic energy is being produced by only the small portion of the vocal folds surrounding the nodules. The anterior and posterior regions fail to close, demonstrating an hourglass configuration. This results in increased breathiness.

B. Nodules

Case 14: Nodules

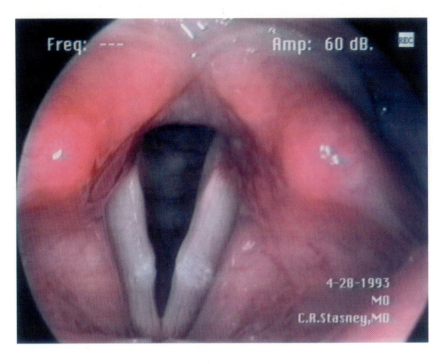

In this instance, the patient, an 18-year-old female student, is an ebullient, extrovert who was a class leader and cheerleader in high school. One sees the typical "hard nodules" at the juncture of the anterior and middle thirds of the vocal folds. One striking difference from the previous example (case 13) is that the nodular swellings are covered with a small amount of leukoplakia (white patch), reflecting their chronicity. Nodules are much like having callouses on the feet from shoes that are too tight; they result from repetitive irritation at the point of maximum impact of the vocal folds. Nodules are more common in the female (or prepubertal male) larynx. They result from chronic vocal abuse in the singing and/or speaking voice. One can appreciate the fact that vocal abuse can be a co-factor with such activities as smoking and acid reflux in the development of cancer of the larynx.

Pathophysiology

These nodular swellings have increased to the size where they are the only contact points during phonation. The hourglass configuration is evident at all times except just prior to phonation when excessive tension of the ventricular folds is used to achieve complete closure. The vibratory source is confined to the nodules and paranodular tissue.

Case 15: Nodules

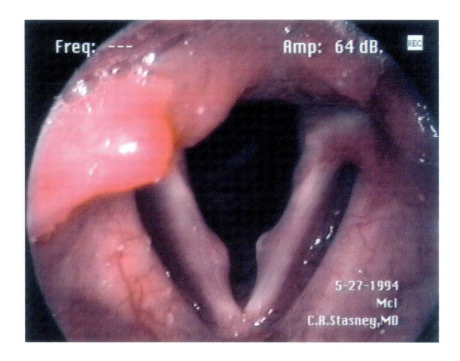

Here one can see the effects of untrained "belting" on the larynx. This 18-year-old female pop singer is a world-class belter and would-be Broadway singer. Some roles lend themselves to vocal abuse, but well-trained Broadway singers have learned how to "belt" without as much strain on the vocal folds.

Pathophysiology

These nodules are significantly interfering with normal vocal fold vibrations. The only vibratory source is the nodules themselves, resulting in a very weak sound with extreme breathiness. (Fig 15)

Case 15 (continued)

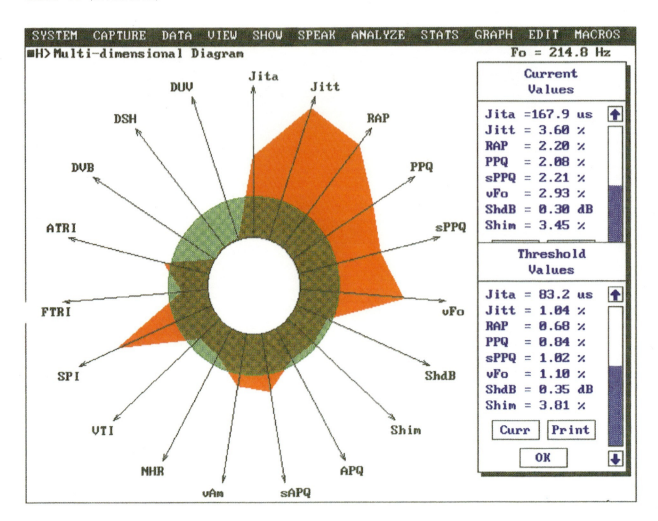

Fig 15

Case 16: Nodules

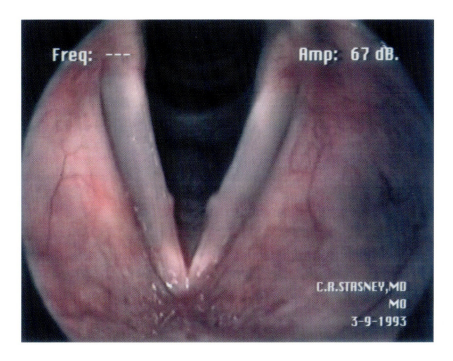

This 30-year-old female soprano (well known to the opera world) has minor irregularities at the typical location on her vocal folds (junction of the anterior and middle thirds of the mobile margins). In spite of these, she has a full vocal range and those listening have difficulty detecting any abnormalities. At a meeting of the Voice Foundation several years ago, the late, eminent laryngologist, Dr. Jim Gould, said that many "world-class" opera sopranos have these irregularities, and it would be unwise to label them as "vocal nodules" when one considers the emotional impact on the singer, especially if they are able to sing their normal tessitura. Dr. Gould coined the term "singer's callouses" to describe these lesions.

Pathophysiology

This sample clearly demonstrates how a singer with nodules can produce relatively normal sound at some pitches. At the high pitches, the nodules are compressed to the point that only the posterior region of the folds produces the sound. During the last sustained sample, the lower pitch begins to involve the vibration of the nodules, resulting in poor vocal quality.

Case 17: Nodules

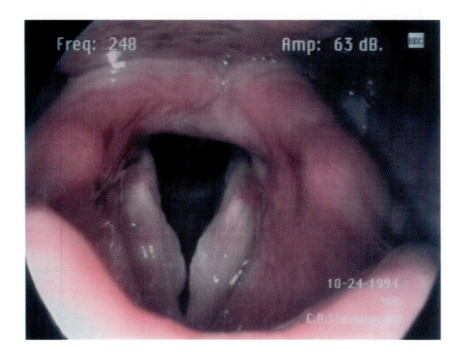

Here one sees broad-based, or sessile, nodules with a white patch (area of leukoplakia) in a 16-year-old female student who is a nonsmoking cheerleader. Obviously, nodules have many forms and the adverse effect on this patient's voice is readily apparent when one listens to her voice sample.

Pathophysiology

The base of each nodule is very large and extends posteriorly. The best vibrations and the best sound are produced at the lower pitches when the vocal folds are lax. The MDD for spoken phonation (Fig 17, a) reveals increased values of frequency and amplitude perturbation from cycle to cycle as well as higher values of SPI (Soft Phonation Index) and VTI (Voice Turbulence Index). As is seen in many cases, this patient exhibited better phonation during sung production (Fig 17, b) than spoken production. There is less frequency perturbation and less noise during sung phonation.

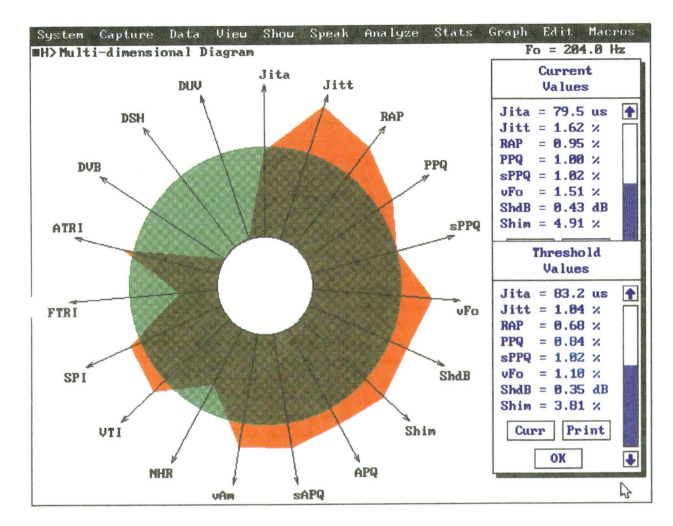

Fig 17A

Case 17 (*continued*)

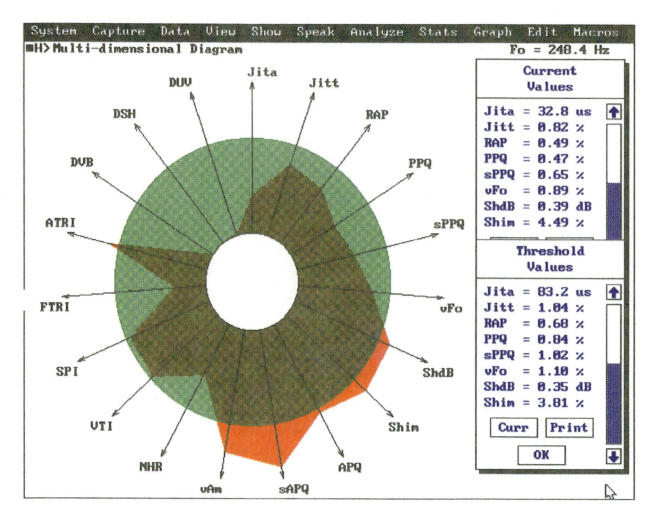

Fig 17B

C. Polyps

The etiology of polyps is open to much debate. Suffice it to say that they are usually the result of hyperfunction and many times occur after a vocal fold hemorrhage. Polyps vary in location and type with the most common types listed below. They are usually unilateral, but may be accompanied by a nodular type lesion on the contact point of the opposite fold. Whereas nodules respond to speech therapy with approximately a 70% improvement, polyps have a much poorer prognosis. Polyps require surgical care around 80% of the time followed by a course of vocal rehabilitation if conservative therapy is unsuccessful.

Case 18: Angiomatous polyp

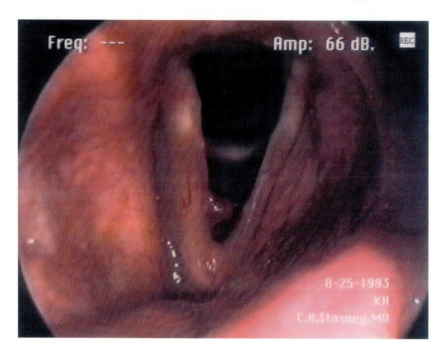

This 60-year-old male politician suffers from an angiomatous polyp. Polyps occur as the result of phonotrauma and are many times secondary to new vessel growth into a segment of the vocal fold (e.g., after a hemorrhage) which becomes persistent. Vocal fold polyps occur much more commonly in the male (73% male vs. female).[1] Kleinsasser states that many polyps originate from ectatic vessels which rupture, then become organized by sprouting capillaries which cause the polyps to grow and take on the appearance of an angioma.[1] These are relatively unresponsive to conservative therapy and generally require surgical removal after appropriate vocal rehabilitation.

Pathophysiology

Polyps have differing effects on vocal fold vibrations, depending on the location and extent of the base as well as the mechanical effects of the mass of the body of the polyp. In this sample, the base of the polyp is located on the vibrating margin of the folds and the mass of the polyp lies directly between the folds. These two factors typically result in the most dramatic reduction in vocal fold vibrations and vocal quality. The posterior region of the unaffected left fold is the primary source for vibrations.

Case 19: Gelatinous polyp

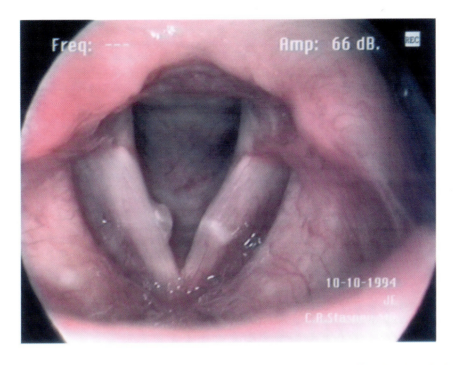

In this case (that of a 22-year-old female congressional staff person), one readily sees the clear, cystic polyp involving the junction of the anterior and middle thirds of the right vocal fold. There is a small contact nodular lesion at a similar site on the opposing fold.

Pathophysiology

Although this sample has a small polyp compared to the other samples, the effect on vocal fold vibrations is significant. The polyp has a wide base attached to the vibrating margin and the mass of the polyp prevents the vocal folds from closing. Perceptually, the voice is characterized by consistent hoarseness with intermittent voice breaks. This case clearly demonstrates the value of the stroboscopy and MDD in understanding the cause of the perceptual characteristics. The hoarseness component is caused by inability of the vocal folds to vibrate synchronously. The offset nature of the vibrations of the two folds results in increased values of pitch and amplitude perturbation on the MDD and the perception of hoarseness. At times the mass of the polyp interferes with the vibration of the opposite fold to the extent that vibration ceases, resulting in the pitch breaks. The MDD pattern (Fig 19) is typical of an individual with hoarseness and voice breaks. The increased values of DSH (Degree of Sub-Harmonic components) and DUV (Degree of Voiceless) are due to the intermittent voice breaks where the regular nature of the fundamental frequency breaks down. The DSH values increase when the multiples of the fundamental frequency are detected and the absence of periodic vibration raises the DUV value.

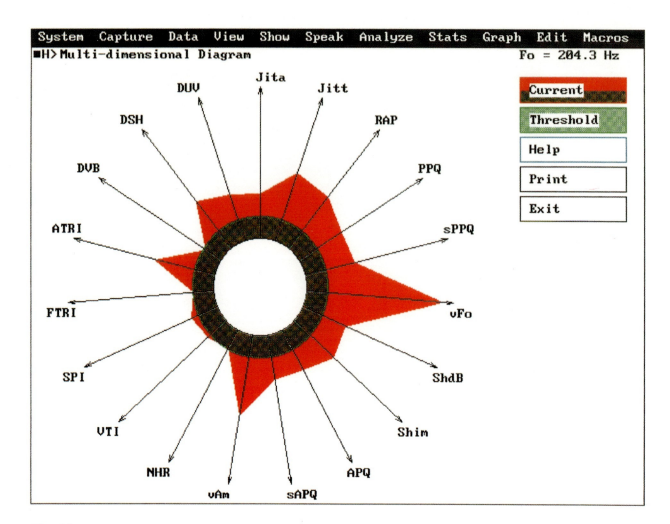

Fig 19

Case 20: Fibrous polyp

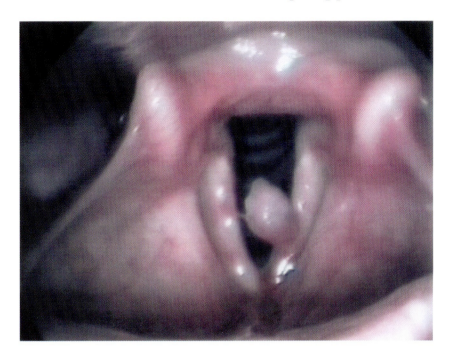

Another example of the plethora of different types of polyp is seen in this 33-year-old female gospel singer. Notice the way in which this lesion is forced above the level of the vocal folds, resulting in much better approximation (and thereby a better voice) than if the polyp stayed at the fold level.

Pathophysiology

This polyp is large but has a thin base that attaches slightly above the vibrating margins of the folds. The effects of this polyp on phonation are variable and are dependent on the location of the major mass of the polyp. At times the polyp itself begins vibrating resulting in the perception of diplophonia (two simultaneous vibrations).

Case 21: Extensive polypoid corditis

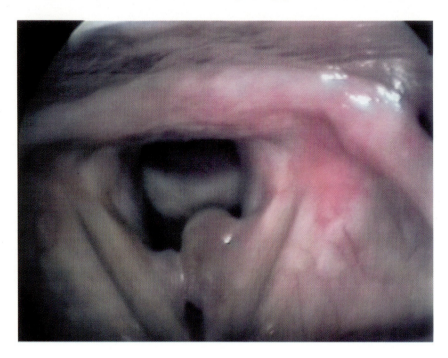

Imagine the larynx of Louis Armstrong! It must have been similar to this. The effect on voicing is evident in this case of a well-known 44-year-old male folk singer. However, he was happy with his voice, and was seen for ear complaints at the office. Obviously, the role of the voice specialist is not always to achieve perfectly straight folds, or an improved range, but to help the singer understand how the larynx works and the way in which to keep his or her voice as healthy as possible for as long as possible.

Pathophysiology

The smaller right polyp attaches directly on the vibrating margin and the larger left polyp is slightly above. The attachment location and the soft nature of the mass allow the polyps to participate in the vocal fold vibrations.

D. Cysts and Laryngoceles

Cysts and laryngoceles have been comingled because of similar histopathology. Both lesions have a lining epithelium (columnar, cuboidal, or squamous), and phonotrauma does not seem to play a role in their development (unlike pseudocysts). This text will refer to laryngoceles and saccular cysts as being of the same ilk. Laryngoceles are merely saccular cysts that still communicate with the airway via a connection in the laryngeal ventricle. Saccular cysts arise from "pinched off" portions of the saccule, contain fluid, and do not communicate with the airway. There are internal and external laryngoceles (the latter extend through the thyrohyoid membrane and the former do not). Laryngoceles, or saccular cysts, may occur as congenital lesions and cause stridor in the newborn.[2]

True cysts are of the ductal or epithelial inclusion variety. Mucous retention cysts (ductal cysts) can occur anywhere there are mucous glands. They result from obstruction of the opening of the glands to mucous membranes. In the elderly population many ductal cysts are made up of oncocytic type cells.[3]

Epithelial inclusion cysts may be congenital or acquired. One hypothesis is that they occur from repeated phonotrauma which drives epithelial cells into the subepithelial tissue. An unusual type of supraglottic cyst is the thyroglossal duct cyst which may present as a supraglottic mass causing dorsiflexion of the epiglottis by filling the preepiglottic space.[4]

Case 22: Saccular cyst

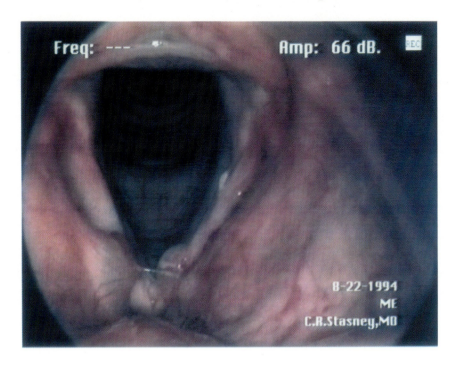

This case, a 37-year-old priest, represents a saccular cyst on the right and a focus of papillomatosis on the left vocal fold. The patient has had numerous recurrences of laryngeal papillomas with multiple surgical procedures. It is possible that the saccular cyst on the right resulted from obstruction of the saccule of the ventricle by either papilloma or scar tissue from papilloma removal.

Pathophysiology

This supraglottic saccular cyst does not appear to interfere with the vocal fold vibrations. The papilloma on the anterior portion of the left fold prevents the anterior portion of the folds from approximating. The persistent gap results in a perceptually breathy quality to the voice.

Case 23: Bilateral internal laryngoceles

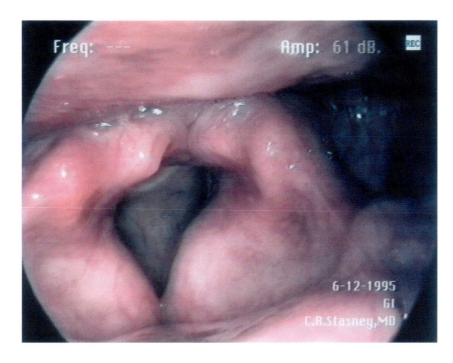

This case is that of an 75-year-old male with bilateral internal laryngoceles. Note the lack of closure of the true folds caused by the "door-stopping" action of the false fold approximation.

Pathophysiology

The extreme size of the ventricular folds prevent any closure of the true folds. The acoustic energy used to speak is primarily the result of air turbulence from air pushed through a posterior chink similar to the production of a loud whisper. Intermittent low frequency vibrations occur when the supraglottic tissue is compressed around the upper region of the chink. This patient uses this extreme form of hyperfunction to compensate for inability to approximate the true vocal folds. Speech treatment to reduce the hyperfunctional muscle activity is an integral part of restoring the voice after surgery.

Case 24: Glottic cyst

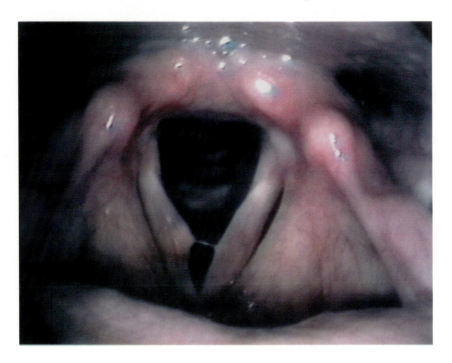

This case, that of a 38-year-old housewife, demonstrates a glottic (intracordal) cyst inside the mass of the right true fold. The yellowish tint of the cyst makes it stand out from the remainder of the fold; however, many times the distinction is not so clear. Cysts can occur in the false or true folds or be associated with the ventricles (as with most laryngoceles).

Pathophysiology

The stiffness and extent of this glottic cyst prevent vibration in the central portion of the folds. The primary vibratory source is the region of the vocal folds anterior to the cyst. The posterior region remains open in the form of a chink contributing to the breathy nature of the voice.

Case 25: Subglottic cyst

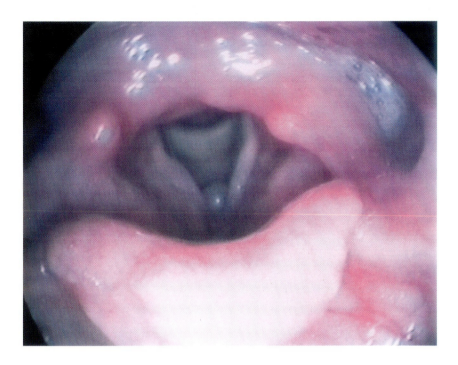

Subglottic cysts may occur as the result of long-term intubation in infants.[5] This particular case is that of a 76-year-old housewife. A cyst is noted in the anterior subglottis which, on histologic examination, proved to be an oncocytic cyst. These usually occur in the elderly patient's supraglottis and result from oncocytic cell proliferation.[6] Of incidental note in this patient is Reinke's edema involving the right vocal fold which results in an inward and downward deflection of the mid-fold mucosa on inspiration and will be discussed in case 28.

Pathophysiology

The anterior subglottic cyst appears to exert a minor amount of upward deflection of the anterior folds. This, combined with the Reinke's edema and tremor, results in a low-pitched raspy voice. Notice how the stroboscopy image frequently fails to trigger appropriately due to the irregularity of the fundamental frequency.

E. Edema

Case 26: Edema secondary to abuse

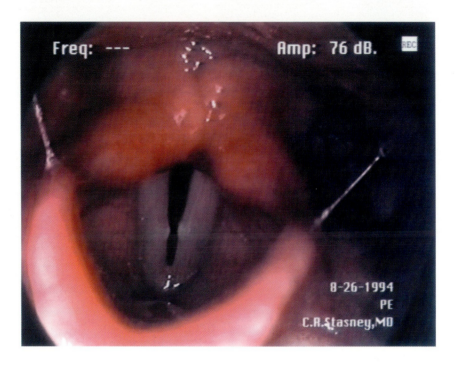

This example is that of a 22-year-old opera singer who has just performed the role of Aida in her college opera production. A slight swelling like this can occur "physiologically" following a vigorous Puccini or Verdi leading soprano role. Generally, these will subside over 24 hours with no treatment and are not usually cause for concern unless the performer must sing again within that time span.

Pathophysiology

This patient's primary complaint was a loss of voicing, 3 to 5 top tones in the upper register following vigorous voice use. The stroboscopy reveals how minor swellings can interfere with vocal fold vibrations at the upper extent of the singing range while having little effect on the speaking voice or singing in the lower part of the range. The upper part of a singer's range is produced by a dramatic lengthening of the vocal folds. The vocal folds become more tense and have less contact area during vibration at high pitches. As the contact area decreases, the swellings take up a higher proportion of the vibrating margin. This results in the greatest amount of interference with vocal fold vibration when singing in the upper range.

Case 27: Reinke's edema

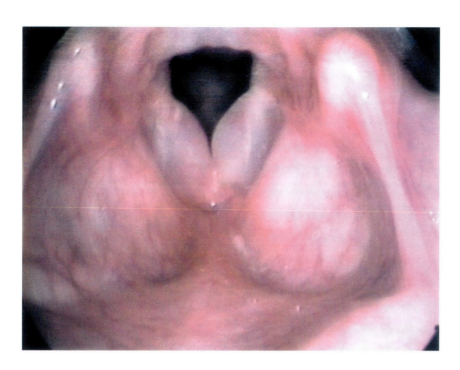

This case of a 58-year-old housewife with a 70 pack-year history of tobacco abuse (calculated by multiplying the number of packs smoked per day by the number of years the person smoked) clearly demonstrates a case of Reinke's edema. Reinke's edema occurs between the superficial and middle layers of lamina propria (Reinke's space). It is more frequent in females than in males and usually is associated with tobacco abuse. Reinke's edema frequently results in loss of high range as mass is added to the vocal folds in the form of viscous material in Reinke's space.

Case 28: Chronic allergy

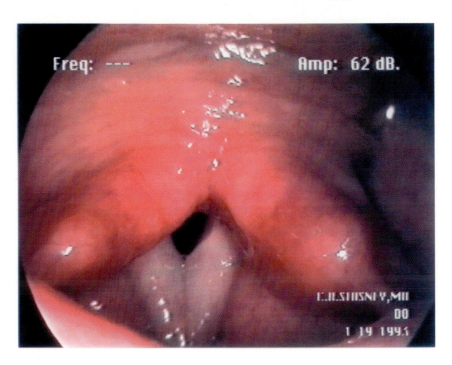

The larynx can be a target organ for an allergic diathesis. This can range from grayish swollen mucosa to edema in Reinke's space, to angioneurotic edema with airway compromise. In the case of this 45-year-old executive secretary, the mild diffuse edema of both folds is apparent, although subtle. This diagnosis is difficult with videostroboscopy and relatively impossible with the mirror. One must remain suspicious, and the history combined with a good stroboscopic exam will facilitate the correct diagnosis.

Case 29: Acute allergy

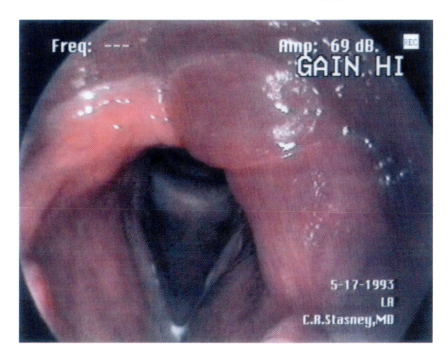

This 29-year-old architect developed acute laryngeal edema following exposure to shellfish (to which he was known to be allergic). Diffuse edema of the left supraglottic larynx, including the left arytenoid, aryepiglottic fold, and false fold are seen in this example.

F. Ulcers and Granulomas

Case 30: Contact ulcer

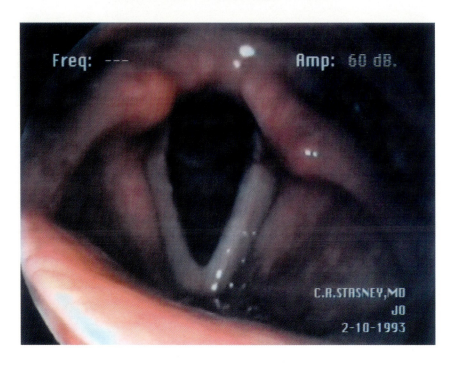

This example of a left contact ulcer is seen in a 38-year-old business executive. Contact ulcers are usually found on the vocal process of one (or both) arytenoid(s). As the vocal process mucosa is very thin, one can imagine the effect of repetitive throat clearing as an etiologic factor. Most patients with contact ulcers and granulomas are male, hard-driven executives who suffer from an oversupply of type A personality. In addition, gastric acid reflux plays an etiologic role in many of these cases.[7] In this case, one readily appreciates the ulcer on the left vocal process and possibly on the right as well.

Pathophysiology

Patients with contact ulcers and contact granulomas frequently exhibit functional behaviors that may either cause or exacerbate the problem. The most common functional problems are excessively loud speech, harsh glottal attacks, and laryngeal hyperfunction with or without excessive neck tension. The most common non-speech functional problems are excessively harsh habitual throat clearing and coughing. The diagnosis and treatment of these functional problems can play an important role in therapy.

Case 31: Contact granuloma

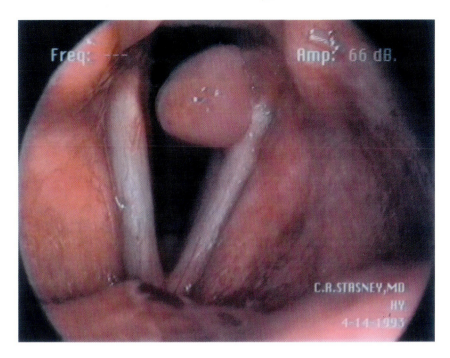

This 67-year-old male retired military officer demonstrates a large contact granuloma of the vocal process of his left arytenoid. Most contact granulomata are unilateral and thought to be secondary to attempts to heal a contact ulcer with a plethora of granulation tissue. A relationship with gastroesophageal reflux and chronic throat clearing is likely. There is even a suggestion to rename the disease "peptic granuloma."[8] Granulomas usually occur on the vocal process of the arytenoid, but may form on other anatomical sites in the larynx. The exact etiology of contact granulomata is imprecisely understood; however, physical and phonotrauma seem to play a role. Airway compromise is possible and a real danger in some of the larger lesions.

Pathophysiology

The long stalk of the base of this granuloma allows the excess tissue to be pushed above the folds during phonation allowing relatively good sound production. The reduction in the quality of phonation is due to the large mass resting on the vocal folds and the inability to completely close the posterior region of the folds.

Case 32: Intubation granulomata

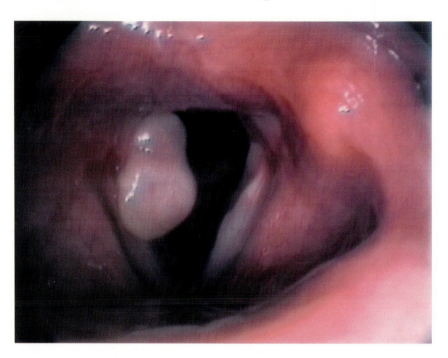

Intubation granulomata usually are bilateral and occur on the vocal processes of the arytenoids. They occur following intubation (generally for extended cases) and have a good prognosis for spontaneous resolution. This 54-year-old housewife, who is 4 weeks post-op major abdominal surgery, has a large granuloma on the right and a very small one on the left vocal process.

Pathophysiology

The effect of this granuloma on phonation is much more severe than the previous case. The granuloma remains directly between the vocal processes of the arytenoids preventing the adduction of the vocal folds. The ensuing large gap results in a breathy voice with short maximum phonation times. To compensate for the obstruction, this patient attempts to phonate by lowering the pitch (to make the folds short and lax) and using extreme anterior-posterior compression, producing a moderately strained vocal quality.

Case 33: Teflon™ granuloma

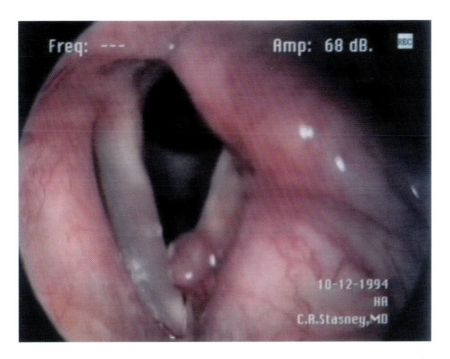

Teflon™ granulomas generally occur many years following a Teflon™ injection and present a therapeutic dilemma. This patient, a 56-year-old food service employee, had a paralyzed left vocal fold following an anterior cervical fusion. The paral-ysis persisted for 1 year and she was injected with Teflon™ 12 years before presenting to the Texas Voice Center with severe dysphonia. The granular-appearing lesion on the superior surface of the left vocal fold and its effect on fold function is apparent.[9]

Pathophysiology

Perceptually, this patient has an extremely raspy voice with diplophonia present. The explanation for the severity of the voice is apparent with the stroboscopy. Due to the effects of the granuloma, nearly two-thirds of the left vocal fold is stiff to the extent that it is adynamic during phonation. The posterior third of the left fold is pliable enough to vibrate and tends to vibrate at its own frequency. The mass of the granuloma also precludes the right fold from vibrating in a regular manner. The result is that the two folds vibrate at different frequencies, precluding any consistent periodicity. When analyzing the acoustic signal, it is important that all information be evaluated. The MDD shows extreme abnormalities in nearly every parameter (Fig 33, a). When these extreme values occur, it is often indicative of vibrations that are aperiodic to the extent that the program is unable to evaluate any consistent regularity to the signal. From examination of the fundamental frequency contour and the F_0 histogram, it is clear that most of the acoustic signal is aperiodic, resulting in no tracking or wildly fluctuating vibrations (Fig 33, b).

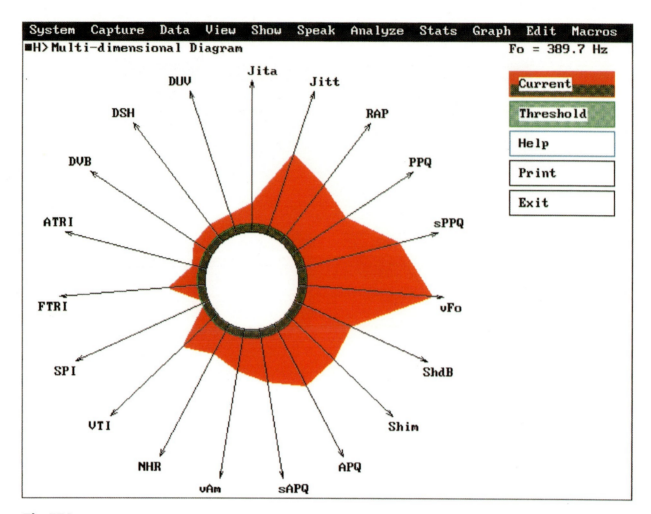

Fig 33A

Case 33 (*continued*)

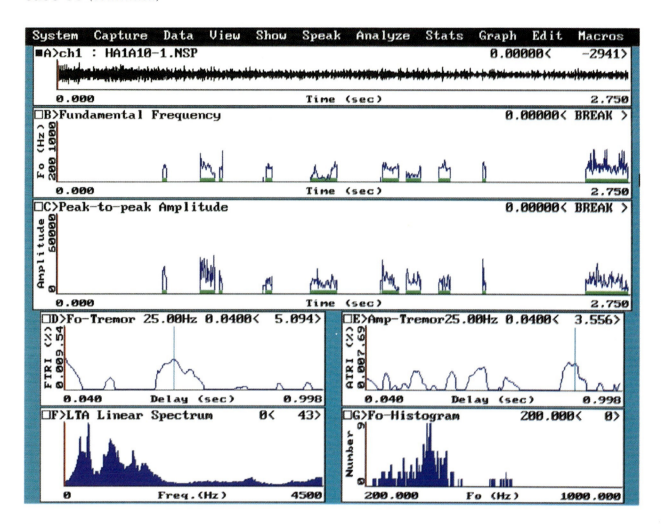

Fig 33B

Case 34: Teflon™ granuloma

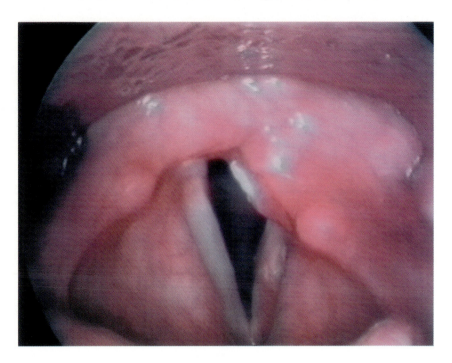

This patient, a 23-year-old female secretary, had a left vocal fold paralysis stemming from an anterior cervical fusion. She was injected with Teflon™ 13 years before presenting to the Texas Voice Center. The injection technique was unknown, but the swollen area immediately above the medial left arytenoid proved to be a foreign body granuloma and apparently the Teflon™ migrated to this location. In addition, the mid portion of the left vocal fold was very firm with an extensive amount of fibrous and granulation tissue with foreign body giant cell proliferation as well.

Pathophysiology

Perceptually the voice has a very breathy component. Visualizing the stroboscopy, the left fold is fairly stiff due to the Teflon™ granuloma; however, the edge is straight allowing the right fold to vibrate against it. The perceptually breathy component is due to the presence of a consistent posterior gap.

Case 35: Wegener's granulomatosis

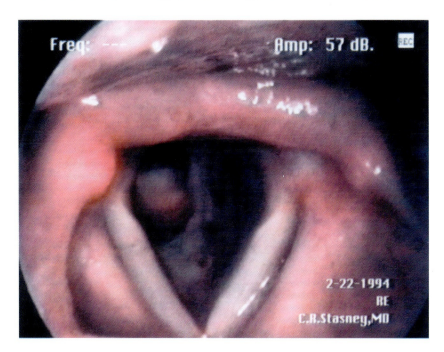

Wegener's granulomatosis is a disease involving a multitude of body systems. The triad of vasculitis, granuloma formation, and necrosis with scar formation involving respiratory ciliated columnar epithelial mucous membranes is the hallmark of this disease. The subglottic trachea is one of the sites of predilection for Wegener's granulomatosis. The vocal folds are relatively spared because they are covered with squamous epithelium. The incidence of subglottic stenosis is approximately 16% of Wegener's granulomatosis patients.[10] In this example, that of a 47-year-old female secretary, the subglottic stenosis with scar formation is apparent, extending from just below the true folds to just above the carina. The patient exhibited biphasic stridor.

G. Inflammation

Case 36: Laryngitis sicca

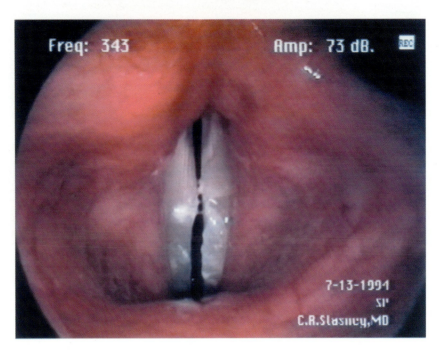

In the case of this 21-year-old musical theater student, the patient graphically demonstrates the effect of viscous mucus on vocal fold function. One can appreciate the tethering effect of the tenacious mucus on the folds as they cycle. The analogy of rubber cement is appropriate to describe the effect of dry sticky mucus on the vocal folds. The psychological benefit of videostroboscopy is wonderful, because once professional voice users see this image, they immediately begin to drink more fluids and increase their hydration.

Pathophysiology

The high viscosity of this patient's mucus combined with it's cohesive nature results in minor changes in vocal fold vibrations, primarily in the lower frequencies. The posterior gap adds a small breathy component, as indicated by a slightly higher Soft Phonation Index (Fig 36, a). Notice the MDD of the sung voice (Fig 36, b). The only parameters outside the normal range are reflective of normal vibrato production. All other parameters are well within normal range. The MDD pattern seen during singing is frequently improved over that of speech. This is most likely due to increased efficiency in the use of the respiratory system resulting in improved periodic vocal fold vibrations as well as better vocal fold closure when singing.

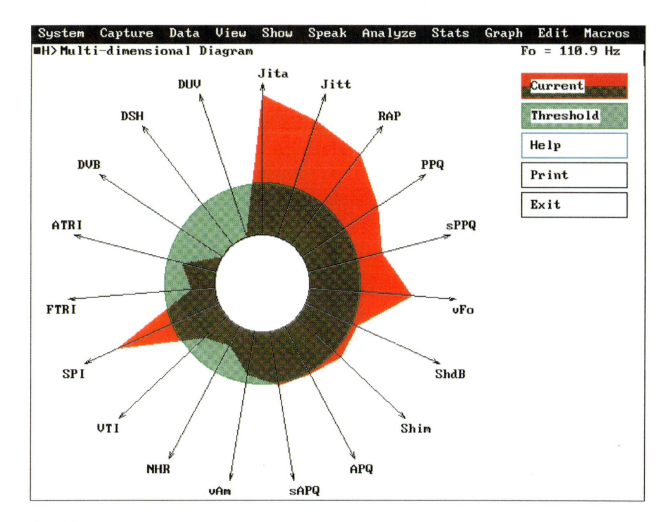

Fig 36A

Case 36 (continued)

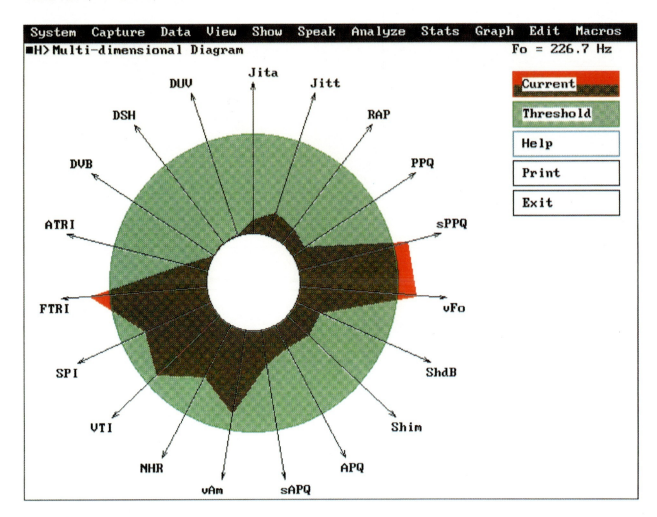

Fig 36B

Case 37: Acute laryngitis

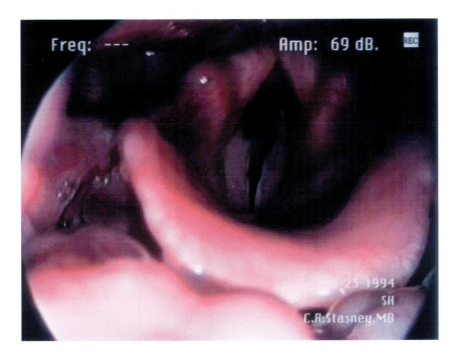

In the case of this 31-year-old male classical singer, the folds are irregularly edematous and fail to approximate in a symmetrical fashion, thereby creating regular, mirror-image oscillations. Here the inflammation is apparent; however, in acute laryngitis, the only manifestation often is diffuse edema.

Pathophysiology

In this patient the vocal processes of the arytenoids are not fully brought together, and there is very little tension in the thyroarytenoid muscles within the vocal folds. This leaves a full gap along the entire length of the vocal folds, preventing phonation from occurring.

Just prior to each time the vocal folds begin vibrating, a minor adjustment of the arytenoids is noticed which places them in the correct configuration for vocalization. This is a common compensatory behavior that occurs when the vocal folds are tender or irritated.

Case 38: Chronic laryngitis

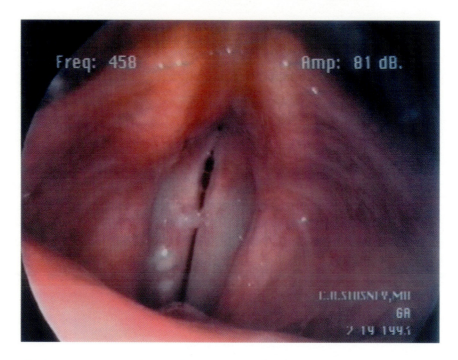

In this 49-year-old business executive with a 60 pack-year tobacco abuse history, the vocal folds are noted to be thickened, relatively adynamic, and with prominent vessels on the dorsal surface. The right fold is particularly inelastic, and the limitation of mucosal wave is apparent.

Pathophysiology

The extremely stiff nature of the right vocal fold results in reduced mucosal waves occurring during high frequencies. At the lower frequencies, the stiff vocal fold does vibrate, but the differences in the stiffness of the two folds results in asynchronous vibrations. During speaking the patient compensates for the adynamic aspects of the right vocal fold by keeping the folds in a short, lax configuration.

Case 39: Chronic laryngitis

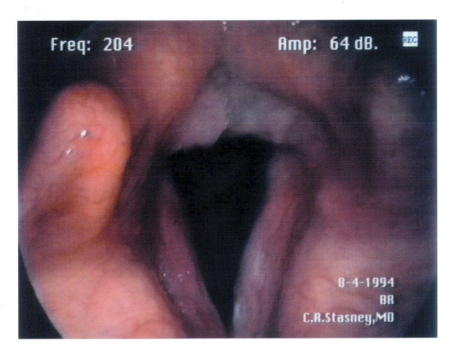

This 40-year-old male rhythm and blues singer had many cofactors which resulted in the devastating appearance of these vocal folds. Reflux of stomach acid (to be discussed more fully regarding the next case), tobacco abuse (he does not smoke but performs in many smoky places and is therefore subject to "second-hand" smoke), and vocal abuse all combine to cause the chronic laryngitis in this patient. An occult malignancy, especially involving the right fold, is possible and these patients need to be carefully watched and the offending cofactors eliminated, if possible.

Pathophysiology

To compensate for the irregular edges of the vocal folds, this patient has attempted to increase the overall activity of the intrinsic laryngeal muscles. Unfortunately, a reverse effect is occurring. There is excessive compression of the arytenoid cartilages as well as excessive anterior to posterior compression. This compression reduces the longitudinal tension of the vocal folds, which in turn decreases the ability of the vibrating margins of the vocal folds, to approximate during phonation.

Case 40: Reflux laryngitis

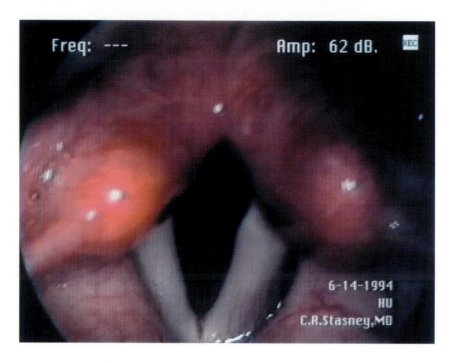

Note the "cherry red" arytenoids in this 42-year-old rehabilitation therapist. Although this is a relatively typical appearance of the larynx with gastroesophageal reflux disease (GERD), there are many other manifestations of the effects of dumping hydrochloric acid and pepsin on the larynx. Contact ulcers and granulomas on the vocal processes of the arytenoids, as well as irritative lesions in other laryngeal sites may be secondary to the effects of GERD.

GERD is underdiagnosed, and clinicians should be suspicious of the possibility when confronted by any of the aforementioned signs and by the following symptoms and diseases: brackish taste in the mouth in the morning, episodic laryngospasm, asthma, chronic throat clearing, heartburn, and dysphonia with the speaking and/or singing voice. The absolute diagnosis is confirmed with two-channel pH probe 24-hour monitoring. We now place the upper pH monitor at the upper part of the upper esophageal sphincter to get a better appreciation of the actual reflux into the hypopharynx and larynx. GERD, if left underdiagnosed and untreated, may lead to serious laryngeal complications including stenoses,[11] reflux laryngitis, globus pharyngeus, carcinoma,[12] and severe respiratory disease.[13] Children are certainly not immune to this disorder, and it has been tied to some cases of chronic bronchitis and laryngitis in children.[14]

Pathophysiology

This patient exhibits some laryngeal behaviors that are a typical response to significant reflux of acid on the posterior portion of the arytenoids and vocal folds. It almost appears as if there is a hesitancy for the arytenoids to come in contact with each other. After voicing, the vocal folds seem to spring apart. This laryngeal behavior is typically unknown and an unconscious behavior on the speaker's part. It is quite possible that this is a protective mechanism organized at a lower level of processing that aids in the preservation of laryngeal tissue.

Case 41: Chemical laryngitis

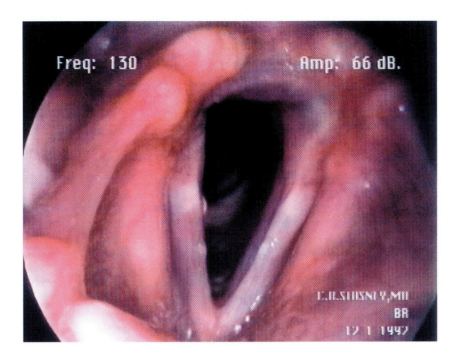

Any form of topical irritation can affect the larynx (as well as the entire tracheobronchial tree). In the case of this 37-year-old pop singer, the patient was exposed to concentrated chlorine vapors as he performed near a swimming pool (there was an explosion with release of chlorine gas). Separating the actual effects from psychological trauma is facilitated by videostrobolaryngoscopy and analysis with the computerized voice lab. Here, one is suspicious of a combination of factors, and the relationship of laryngeal function and psychological overlay is always a relative enigma. Several organic factors appear in the videostroboscopy that deserve comment. The folds are slightly reddened with thick, tenacious mucus. A small gap exists at the juncture of the anterior third of the folds, and there appears to be the beginning of a sulcus on the left fold.

Pathophysiology

One of the most common responses following laryngeal trauma of this nature is that following the trauma, the patient becomes more aware of his voice and changes the way he uses his voice in order to "protect the voice." It is common for people to attempt to protect the voice by reducing the overall amount of effort used to produce voicing. Patients often exhibit this voicing behavior when they are using the "I'm sick" or "I'm tired" voice. Unfortunately, the way phonation is produced is to reduce the amount of respiratory support which in turn reduces the subglottic pressure making the vocal folds vibrate less efficiently.

Case 42: Syphilis

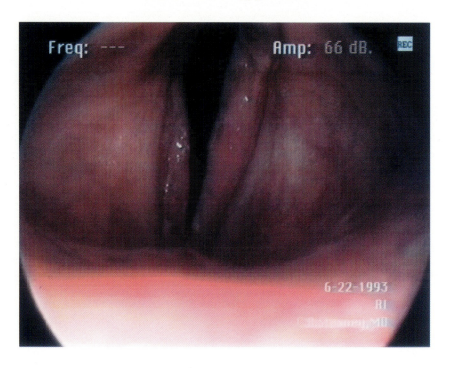

"Know syphilis and tuberculosis and you know Medicine" was time-honored advice given most medical students 50 years ago. It is still sage food for thought as cases 42 and 43 demonstrate. Lues (syphilis) can mimic cancer, Wege-ner's, etc. In this case of a 47-year-old unemployed male, the larynx is red, thickened, with a swollen and immobile left vocal fold. On dark field examination, spirochetes were apparent, and after appropriate medical treatment, the larynx reverted toward a more normal appearance with return of movement of the heretofore immobile fold.

Important to the diagnosis are the serologic studies including the RPR (Rapid Plasma Reagin) and the FTAAbs (Fluorescent Treponemal Antibody Absorption) tests. The former will indicate an acute case whereas the latter will demonstrate that the patient has had an infection in the past (and, therefore, may have congenital lues).[15]

Pathophysiology

The result of this pathology has been increased stiffness along the entire extent of the vocal folds. The posterior half of the left vocal fold is enlarged and is much stiffer. This portion of the left fold does not participate in the vibrations during high pitched vocalizations. During low frequency vocalizations, the difference in the stiffness between the anterior and posterior portions of the left fold results in vibrations that are wildly erratic, accounting for the extremely hoarse nature of the voice during speaking.

Case 43: Tuberculosis

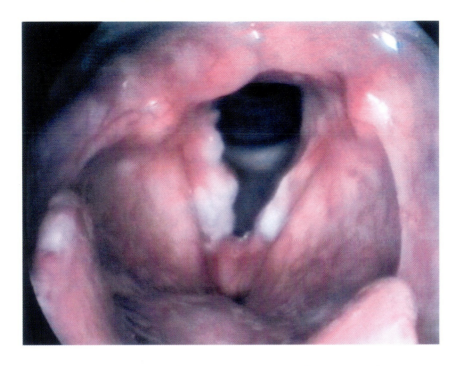

Here's the second half of "knowing medicine." The red, thickened irregular vocal folds covered with blobs of ivory-yellow exudate result in significant dysphonia in this 63-year-old missionary.

Although uncommon, laryngeal tuberculosis is extremely infectious and becoming more prevalent with the rising number of AIDS patients.[16] The vast majority of cases of laryngeal tuberculosis have active pulmonary disease as well. Other fungal infections of the larynx may have a similar appearance. The diagnosis is established by finding the organisms in an acid-fast smear, skin testing, and by demonstrating the caseating granulomas and organisms on histologic exam. Although the folds are relatively mobile in this patient, laryngeal tuberculosis is one of the most frequent causes of recurrent laryngeal nerve paralysis along with malignant neoplasms of the lung.[17] Tuberculosis and syphilis can mimic neoplasia.

Pathophysiology

The right vocal fold is an extreme example of an irregular vocal margin. This sample demonstrates that clear phonation is nearly impossible when the shape of the vibrating margins is highly irregular.

Case 44: Supraglottitis

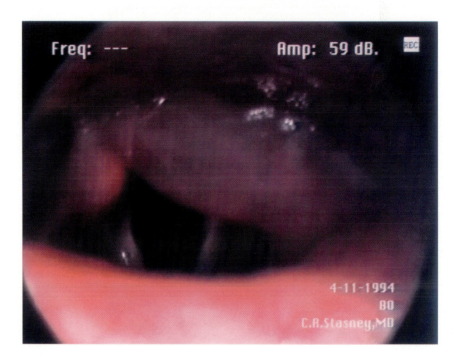

Acute supraglottitis (epiglottitis) occurs in adults as well as in infants and children. The diagnosis is suspected whenever there is a severe sore throat (especially when the patient cannot swallow their own secretions) and confirmed by mirror or fiberoptic examination of the epiglottis. In this case of a 54-year-old housewife, general redness and swelling of the supraglottic structures (particularly the lingual surface of the epiglottis and the left aryepiglottic fold and arytenoid) are apparent. This can be a cause of abrupt airway compromise. The mucosa on the lingual surface of the epiglottis is more loosely attached than that on the laryngeal surface, and this anatomical fact results in a dorsiflexion of the epiglottis with secondary airway obstruction.

Case 45: Arytenoiditis

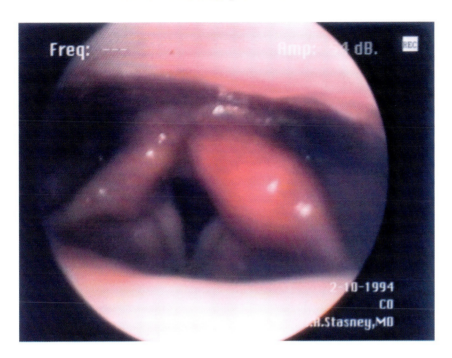

The larynx can be involved with inflammation, infection, and allergic edema (or a combination of all three). In this case of a 55-year-old female housewife, the left arytenoid was swollen in this febrile patient and responded quite nicely to a course of antibiotics and steroids. One must remain suspicious of GERD and allergic etiologies if these lesions recur.

H. Vascular Pathologies

Case 46: Hemorrhage

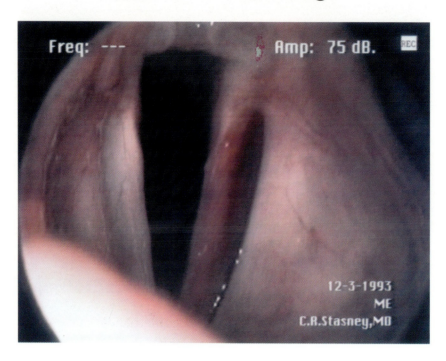

This 50-year-old pop singer suffered from an upper respiratory infection when she tried to belt out all the notes of a popular song and instead caused a rupture in microvessels on the left fold. The situation was exacerbated in this individual because she routinely took an aspirin per day. This may prophylax the heart, but the side effect (of a laryngeal bleed), if it occurs, can be a disaster for the singing voice. One appreciates the diminished mucosal wave on the involved left fold. The increase in mass of the left fold resulted in a loss of high notes and early vocal fatigue. Sometimes, in attempting to effect resolution of the hemorrhage, the body sends in emissary vessels which become relatively permanent and result in an angiomatous polyp. Thereafter, subsequent hemorrhages are more likely, especially if the angiomatous polyp is on the phonating margin of the fold.[18]

Case 47: Varicosities

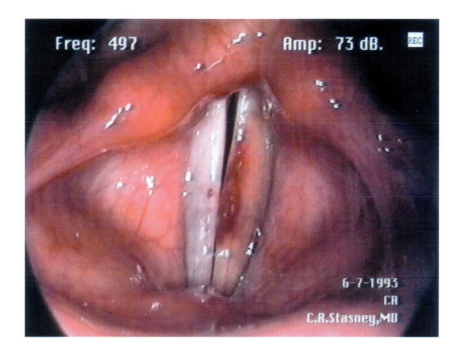

In the case of this 44-year-old female classical singer, varicosities are apparent on the dorsal surface of both vocal folds. There is a resolving hemorrhage on the left fold with what appears to be a forming angiomatous polyp at the juncture of the anterior and middle thirds. Sometimes, these varicosities swell with phonotrauma and may be an etiology for vocal fatigue and loss of range in some patients.

Pathophysiology

This patient demonstrates how one good vocal fold is capable of producing a perceptually clear voice with the absence of abnormal acoustic parameters. Viewing the stroboscopy demonstrates that the affected vocal fold is stiff and participates very little in the vocal fold vibrations. The reason clear voicing can occur is that the stiff affected vocal fold has a straight margin, allowing the healthy fold to produce periodic vibrations that are consistent from cycle to cycle. This points out an interesting observation—the cycle-to-cycle variation seems to produce a much more dramatic effect on the perceived hoarseness than the shape of the waveform itself.

V. VOCAL FOLD CONCAVITY

Case 48: Sulcus

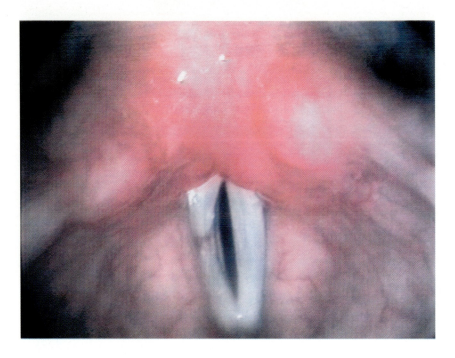

This patient, a 35-year-old female orchestra conductor, has moderate dysphonia secondary to the divot at the juncture of the anterior and middle thirds on the right vocal fold. Some prominent laryngologists feel this lesion occurs at the site of an open epidermoid cyst and that, in effect, it results from spontaneous marsupialization of these cysts.[19]

Pathophysiology

One requirement for synchronous vibration of the vocal folds is that at some point during each cycle the vocal folds must come in contact with each other. The amount of time that the vocal folds are in contact with each other is extremely short; however, the contact time is critical for ensuring synchronization of the two folds so that they will vibrate in phase with one another. The sulcus on the right vocal fold of this patient extends along the entire extent of the vocal fold which prevents the vocal folds from coming in contact with one another during any portion of the vocal fold cycle. The lack of synchronization produces a mildly hoarse voice because the two vocal folds vibrate out of phase and at different rates from each other. The breathy component is also due to the consistent flow of air through the gap.

Case 49: Trough ("vergeture")

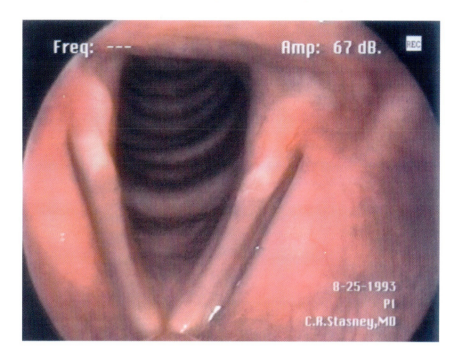

This 65-year-old retired executive demonstrates bilateral true fold troughs (or vergetures). The bilateral troughs are one form of presbylaryngis and may result from atrophy of the structures making up the vocal fold. They also can occur as a congenital lesion and have been termed "vergetures" by Dr. Marc Bouchayer.[20]

Pathophysiology

This patient is similar to the previous patient in that there is a consistent gap between the vocal folds. However, the gap does not extend along the entire length of the vocal folds, thereby allowing some synchronicity to occur by the vibrations that occur at the anterior and posterior portions of the vocal folds. The gap is not nearly as wide as in the previous case. These factors result in a voice that is less hoarse and less breathy than the previous patient.

Case 50: Presbylaryngis

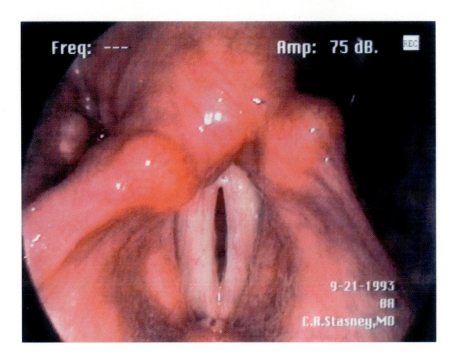

This case of a 66-year-old male judge demonstrates the classic appearance of bowed vocal folds. The question of why this occurs in so many elderly patients and results in a classic dysphonia so typical of this population is being aggressively investigated by a team at the Van Lawrence Voice Institute at Baylor College of Medicine in Houston. Hopefully, this study will determine exactly what happens to the muscle, mucosa, connective tissue, and joints.

Pathophysiology

A number of factors contribute to the classic dysphonia that is exhibited by so many of the elderly population. These include the reduction of tissue within the vocal folds and/or the lack of tonic muscle activity within the thyroarytenoid muscles which results in the bowing effect seen in this patient. Another important but often overlooked functional factor is a frequent reduction in the strength or ability of the respiratory system. Frequently, patients with minor bowing of the vocal folds due to presbylaryngis can achieve a much clearer voice by increasing the subglottic pressure. An increase in subglottic pressure drives the vocal folds apart with more force during the opening phase of the cycle. During the closing phase, the elasticity of the tissue springs the vocal folds back to the midline with more force, often allowing complete closure to occur during each vocal fold cycle. This greatly improves the quality of the voice.

VI. TRAUMATIC PATHOLOGY

Case 51: Bilateral hematoma

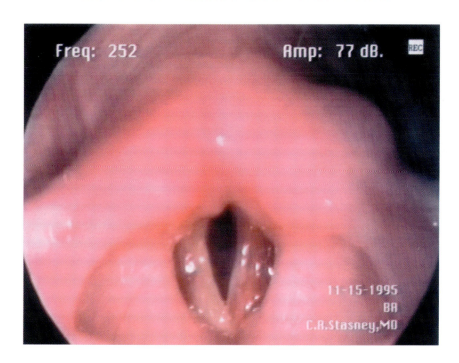

Here is another cause of vocal fold hemorrhage. In this case the 10-year-old male patient was elbowed in the neck while playing basketball. Both vocal folds are involved and care must be taken to check for asymmetry of the folds with disruption of the thyroid cartilage. CT scans often are valuable for additional information.

Case 52: Fracture

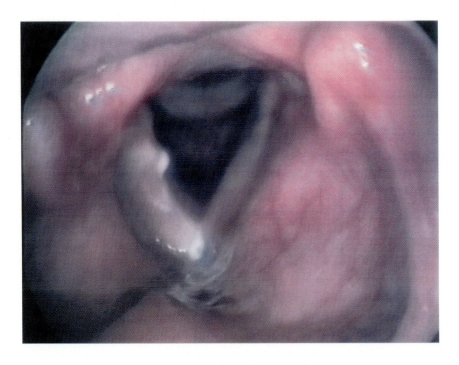

This 30-year-old male engineer was struck in the neck by a hockey puck seven years before this videostroboscopy. Observation was the only therapy reported by the patient, and a possible consequence of the lack of surgical exploration is apparent. The patient is moderately dysphonic, and the right fold appears foreshortened with an anteriorly located right arytenoid and a right vocal process that protrudes somewhat into the airway with a concave right fold. One can only speculate what the result would have been if the patient had undergone emergency exploration with open reduction and fixation of any defects.

Case 53: Torn cord

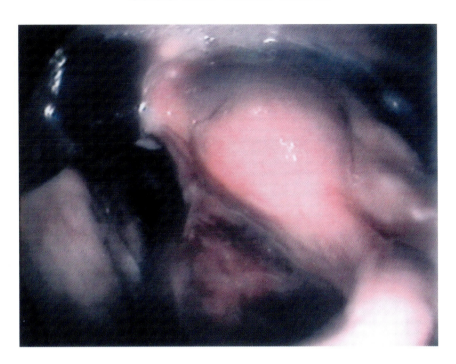

This 38-year-old male construction worker was struck in the throat 6 days before seeking medical attention. The distorted larynx with the hematoma of the left aryepiglottic fold and clot draped over the right arytenoid is apparent. A CT scan, if the airway permits, would give valuable additional information in this patient prior to surgical exploration. Obviously, maintaining an airway is the first priority of the surgeon.

VII. SCARRING OF THE LARYNX

A. Webs

Case 54: Anterior web

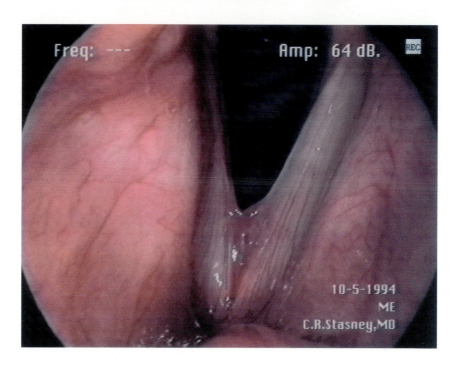

This 62-year-old retired executive became dysphonic 18 months before he was seen in the Texas Voice Center (TVC). A right vocal paralysis was diagnosed and a right thyroplasty was performed 8 months after the dysphonia onset at a major medical center in New York. He persisted with dysphonia and came to the TVC for a second opinion. The paralyzed right vocal fold is apparent, as is a 35% web involving the anterior folds. Whether this web preceded the thyroplasty or not cannot be ascertained by review of New York records. In any case, this patient presents a therapeutic challenge, and the combined effects of the two major pathologies (paralysis and web) are devastating to this patient's voice.

Laryngeal webs are either congenital or acquired and can involve any part of the larynx. Prevention, if possible, is the hallmark of this disease.[21] The next case demonstrates yet another location for a web.

Pathophysiology

The effect of this web on the vibrations of the left vocal fold is extremely interesting. The greatest tethering effect of the web is in the central portion of the vocal folds, producing a left fold in which the anterior and posterior portions of the vocal fold vibrate out of phase with one another (Fig 54).

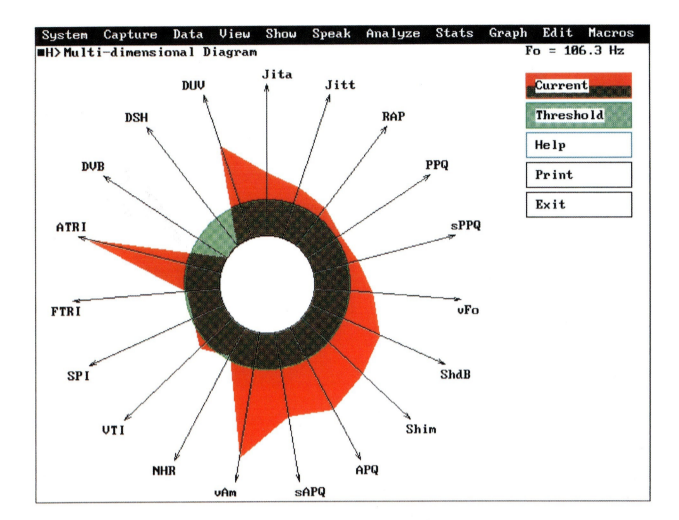

Fig 54

Case 55: Posterior web

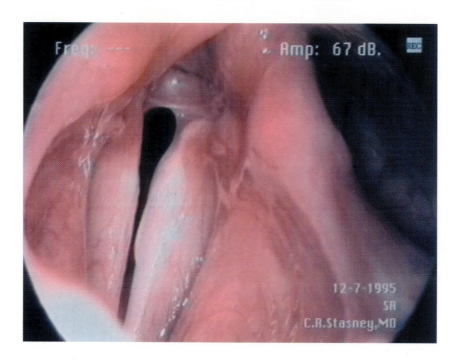

This 14-year-old male student had respiratory complications shortly after birth necessitating prolonged (over 3 months) intubation. When reviewing the videostroboscopy, one notes the limited airway with the tethering effect of the web between the arytenoids. This patient underwent a 24-hour two-channel pH probe esophageal reflux study which demonstrated significant reflux into the oropharynx. Reflux was a possible co-factor in development of the web and was an important therapeutic issue after the web was lysed to prevent recurrence.

Case 56: Anterior web

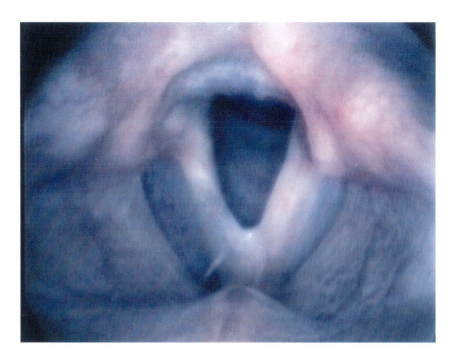

The case of this 43-year-old male executive graphically demonstrates one of the complications of microlaryngeal surgery—web formation following nodule excision. The patient underwent laser nodule removal 4 years prior to his first visit to the Texas Voice Center. One can only speculate regarding the etiology of the web, but one of the most common causes is excision of mucosa too near the anterior commissure bilaterally. Another complication of laser vocal fold surgery, in cases we have reviewed, is scar tissue in the vocal fold with adynamic segments. Needless to say, prevention is the most important factor to be learned from this case. One can readily see the tethering effect of the web on the vocal folds.

Case 57: Anterior web

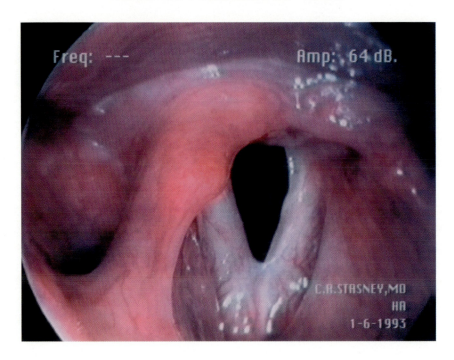

This 61-year-old housewife with Ehlers-Danlos syndrome developed a laryngeal web after esophageal dilatation for idiopathic esophageal stricture. The exact pathogenesis of the abnormality is unknown, but one can infer a relationship with the congenital connective tissue disorder plus the esophageal instrumentation. Webs have a definite relationship to gastroesophageal reflux. Although this patient has reddened arytenoids, she did not have a 24-hour pH monitor to make a definitive diagnosis.

Pathophysiology

The thickness of the tissue joining the anterior portions of the vocal folds is so extensive that it prevents any vibrations from occurring in the anterior portion of the vocal folds. The result of this web is essentially that the effective length of the vibrating vocal folds is reduced by approximately one half of the entire length of the folds. Because the effective length of the vibrating vocal folds is so short, the pitch is dramatically increased.

B. Stenosis

Case 58: Glottic stenosis

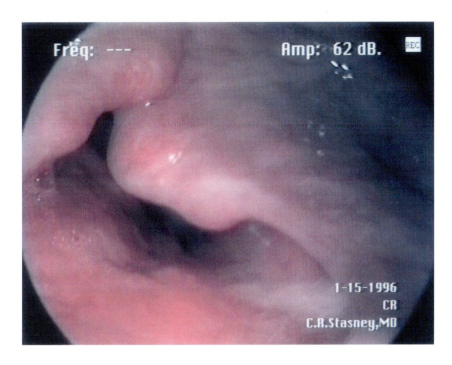

This case demonstrates the resilience of children. The patient is a 10-year-old female who was involved in an automobile accident 5 years prior to her visit to the Texas Voice Center. She suffered laryngeal stenosis, probably secondary to prolonged intubation for a severe head injury. Many procedures were done to open her airway including a cricoid split with bone graft anteriorly. This resulted in an adequate airway, but "railroad track" vocal folds which do not meet anteriorly or posteriorly. This young girl learned to speak using her own particular innovation—she opposes her epiglottis and left corniculate cartilage to elicit oscillation and a mucosal wave. One wonders if this will persist after puberty when the larynx increases in anterior-posterior dimension?

Pathophysiology

The acoustic analysis and perception of the voice are quite good (Fig 58) given the method this patient is using for phonation. The acoustic parameters and perception of this patient's voice are a much higher quality than typically found with patients who use supralaryngeal tissue while voicing.

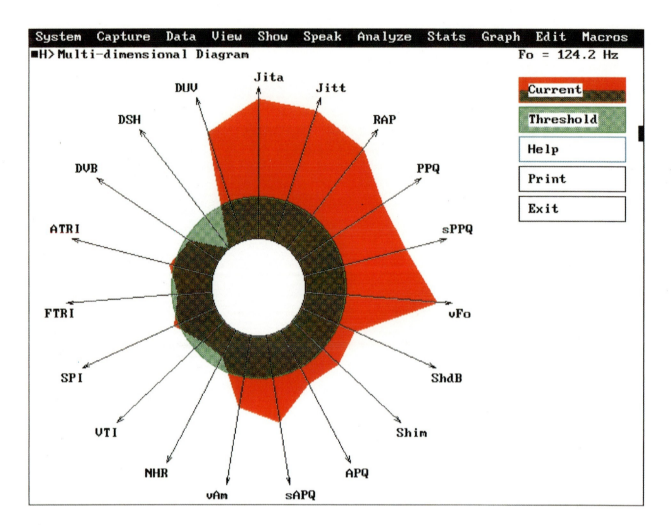

Fig 58

Case 59: Glottic stenosis

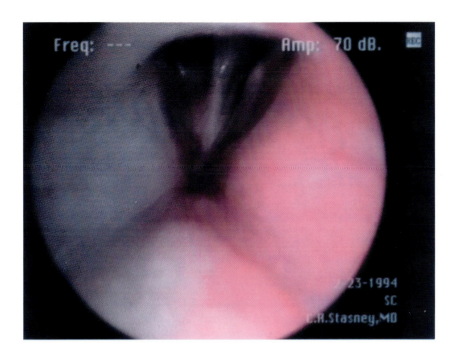

This 16-year-old male student has a story very similar to the previous case, but his stenosis was due to prolonged intubation following a surgical procedure to diagnose lymphoblastic lymphoma which resulted in a severed phrenic nerve at age 6. His laryngeal stenosis was corrected with a cricoid/thyroid cartilage split and rib interposition graft 8 years prior to his visit to the Texas Voice Center. He has "railroad track" vocal folds, but does not compensate as well as the previous case, perhaps because of the larger size of his larynx, and, therefore, the increased distance from his right corniculate cartilage to his epiglottis.

Case 60: Subglottic stenosis

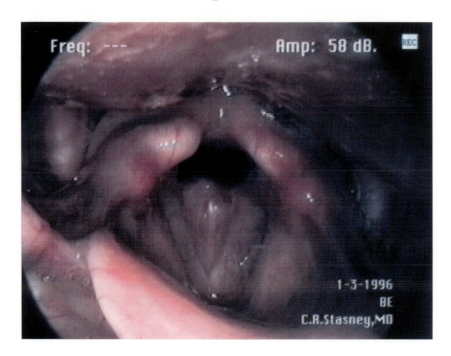

This 38-year-old executive suffers from Epidermolysis bullosa dystrophica. Basically, in this inherited disorder, the epithelial elements separate easily and scar is formed with even minor trauma.[22] The dystrophic form involves separation of the epidermis deep in the basement membrane and more commonly affects the mouth, larynx, and genito-urinary tract.[23] He has undergone many urological procedures for meatal stenosis, unfortunately using endotracheal intubation in each case. The most likely etiology for the laryngeal web is the repeated instrumentation of the larynx by the endotracheal tube. The patient has a weak, high-pitched voice and a marginal airway. One can easily visualize the anterior web extending from the phonating margins of the vocal folds (just anterior to the vocal processes) down to the base of the conus elasticus.

C. Adynamic Vocal Fold Segment

Case 61: Adynamic vocal fold segment

This 60-year-old minister underwent laser microlaryngoscopy for "hemorrhagic polyps" several years before presenting to the Texas Voice Center. His dysphonia is apparent, and even though the vocal folds have a relatively normal appearance when abducted, the adynamic right vocal fold is easily seen on stroboscopy. As with many disorders, prevention is best.

Pathophysiology

An adynamic cord segment typically refers to a portion of the vocal fold that does not participate in vocal fold vibration. The most common cause for this is when the mucosal tissue and/or the vocal fold tissue under the mucosa at the vibrating margin is extremely stiff.

D. Vocal Fold Notching

Case 62: Vocal fold notching

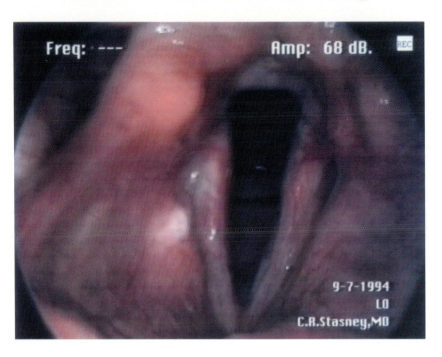

This 30-year-old male professional football coach underwent laser excision for "vocal nodules" 1 year prior to his first visit to the Texas Voice Center. He is unable to project his voice and has significant breathy dysphonia. On stroboscopic examination, the concave folds are apparent with diffuse redness. One can only speculate regarding the preoperative appearance and co-factors (e.g., GERD) that may be involved, but, once again, prevention is the hallmark.[24]

Pathophysiology

Perceptually this patient has a hoarse voice with a breathy component. The stroboscopy demonstrates that the vocal fold notching prevents the main portion of the vocal folds from coming in contact with each other. As discussed previously, the lack of any closed phase during any vocal fold cycle results in the inability of the vocal folds to synchronize. As seen on the MDD (Fig 62), this results in vocal fold vibrations that vary in frequency and amplitude from cycle to cycle. The higher values of SPI (Soft Phonation Index) and VTI (Voice Turbulence Index) are indicative of the persistent gap that is present during phonation. The turbulence of the air flowing through this gap increases the amount of high energy noise which increases these parameters and results in the breathy component.

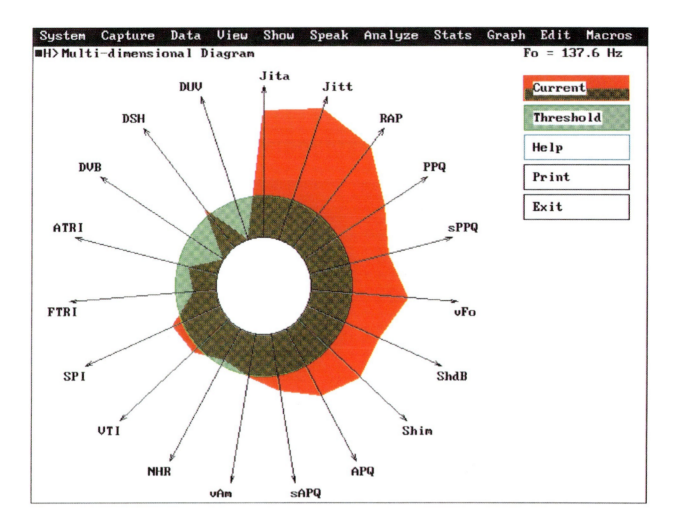

Fig 62

VIII. TUMORS

A. Benign

Case 63: Papillomatosis

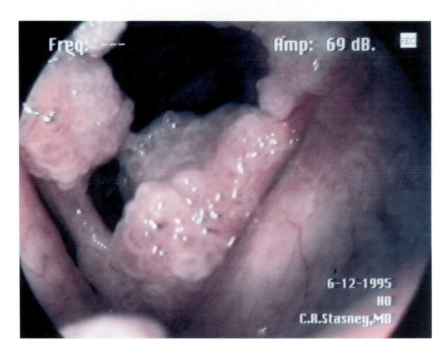

This case graphically demonstrates the aggressive nature of laryngeal papillomatosis. The cauliflower-like profusion of these wart-like fronds from almost every site in the endolarynx (including her epiglottis, posterior commissure, and both true folds) has certainly caused dysphonia, and her airway is marginal. The patient is a 23-year-old secretary who had undergone microlaryngoscopy with laser papilloma excision on two occasions in the year before presenting to the Texas Voice Center.

Papillomatosis, caused by the human papillomavirus types 6, 11, 16, and 18,[25] is an aggressive, recurrent disease which is idiosyncratically responsive to many types of therapy. There is an association with maternal vaginal condylomata in juvenile laryngeal papillomatosis cases. The natural course of the disease is for recurrence; however, sometimes there is spontaneous resolution, and in 2% of cases there is progression to carcinoma.[26]

Pathophysiology

The severity of this patient's papillomatosis prevents any portion of the vocal folds from participating in vibrations. The whisper-like quality of the voice sample is due to this patient's means of phonation. Her sound source is produced by blowing air through a small gap in the posterior region of the folds similar to the configuration produced during a whisper. The air rushing through the small chink produces turbulence in the airstream and creates high frequency noise. Acoustic analysis (Fig 63) simply confirmed that no vocal fold vibrations were present and the signal was made up primarily of high frequency noise.

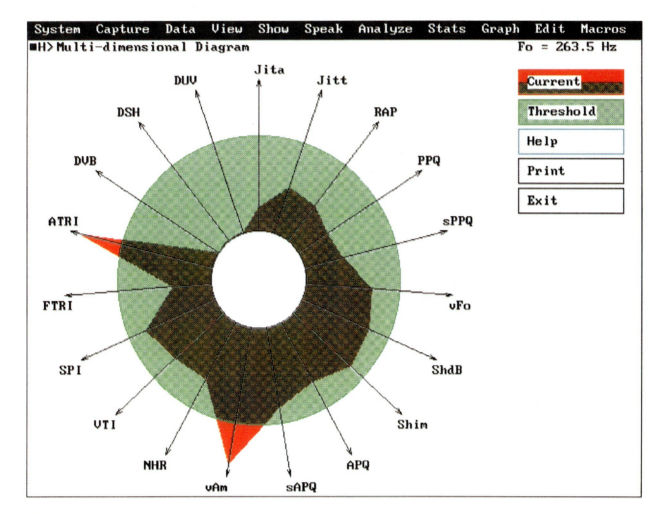

Fig 63

Case 64: Papillomatosis

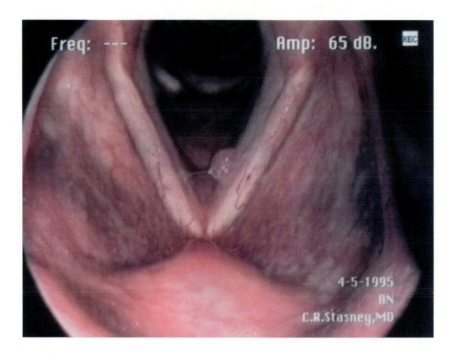

This 50-year-old clinical social worker with a 50 pack-year tobacco abuse history presented with dysphonia and the left vocal fold lesion noted on videostroboscopy. The impact on his vocal function is easily apparent; however, the differential diagnosis would include squamous cell carcinoma, polyp, verrucous carcinoma, and papillomatosis. A mild bilateral vocal fold trough is also apparent when the patient abducts his folds. Microlaryngeal phonosurgery proved the diagnosis of laryngeal papillomatosis.

Pathophysiology

The most significant effect on phonation is produced by the mass of this lesion preventing the vocal folds from achieving closure. As seen on the MDD (Fig 64), this results in short-term and long-term cycle-to-cycle irregularities of the pitch periods. The increased value of SPI is also indicative of the consistent gap that occurs due to the mass occupying lesion.

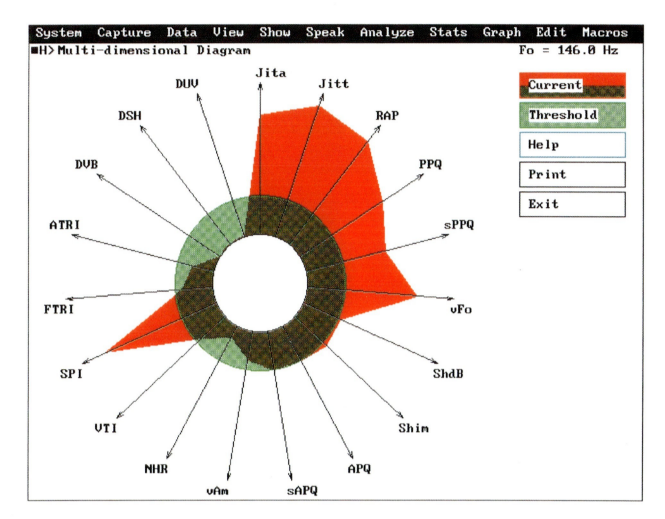

Fig 64

Case 65: Sarcoidosis

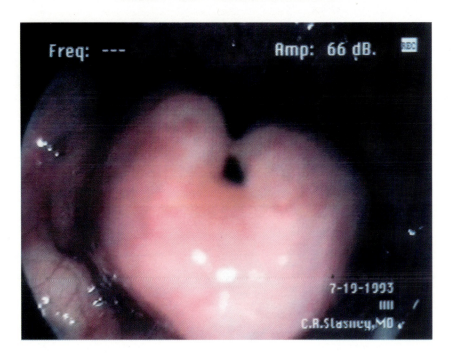

This 40-year-old manual laborer demonstrates the hallmark of laryngeal sarcoidosis, the pale, swollen epiglottis; and he presents with the typical symptoms of dysphonia, dyspnea, and dysphagia.[27]

If these patients develop a viral pharyngitis and present to the otolaryngologist complaining of odynophagia (and they have not been previously seen and diagnosed as sarcoidosis), they may be falsely labeled epiglottitis and taken to the Intensive Care Ward posthaste. Galvan describes the characteristic "honking voice and edematous, pink, diffuse turban-like enlargement of the supraglottic structures."[28] Sarcoidosis is a multiple system disease with frequent exacerbations and remissions. Histopathologically, the lesions are noncaseating granulomata. The diagnosis is based on history, physical examination, and histopathology.

B. Premalignant (hyperkeratosis and leukoplakia)

Case 66: Hyperkeratosis and leukoplakia

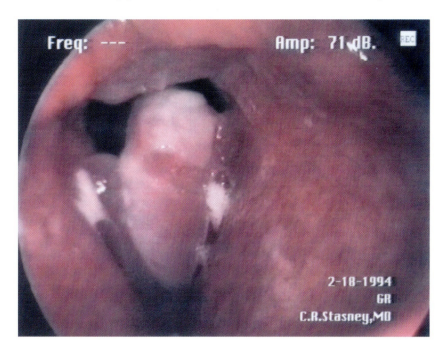

This 51-year-old executive with a 90 pack-year tobacco abuse history demonstrates the image that causes one to think neoplasia when reviewing the videostobic exam. He underwent microlaryngoscopy at which time deep and extensive biopsies were taken. These were reviewed with the pathologist and showed only severe dysplasia, but the patient was encouraged to eliminate tobacco, guard against gastroesophageal reflux, and return for careful follow-up with the admonition that carcinoma might well ensue if he did not cease etiologic co-factors.

Case 67: Hyperkeratosis and leukoplakia

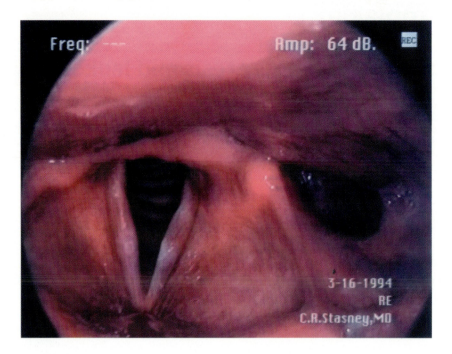

The bilateral mid-fold leukoplakia with Reinke's edema and diminished mucosal wave is apparent in this 49-year-old executive with a 30 pack-year tobacco history. The appearance of the videostroboscopic examination and a careful education of the patient regarding progression to squamous cell carcinoma works wonders in many patients in encouraging them to throw their cigarettes away. It is easy to depersonalize oneself from the dangers of tobacco abuse until one is faced with pulmonary function studies and a video examination of one's own larynx.

Pathophysiology

The MDD (Fig 67) demonstrates that the patient has irregularities of both the short-term and long-term variability of the pitch and amplitude. The failure of the arytenoids to approximate during phonation results in intermittent breakdown of the vocal fold vibrations where the fundamental frequency cannot be detected increasing the DUV (Degree of Voiceless). The tremor seen in the stroboscopic image results in a low frequency amplitude tremor increasing the ATRI (Amplitude Tremor Related Index).

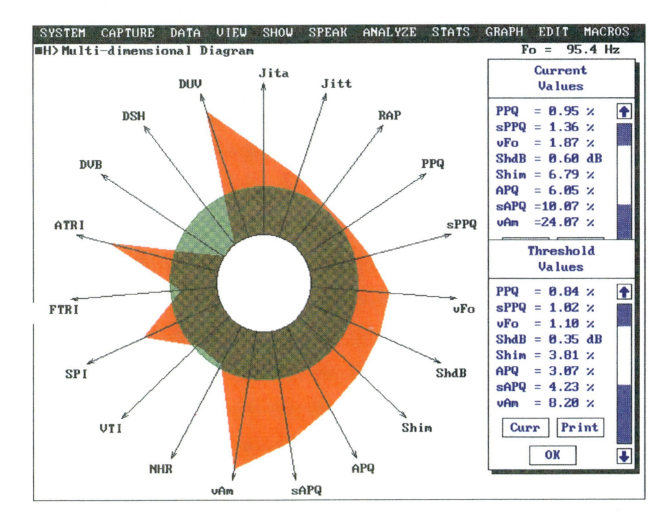

Fig 67

C. Malignant

Case 68: Carcinoma-in-situ

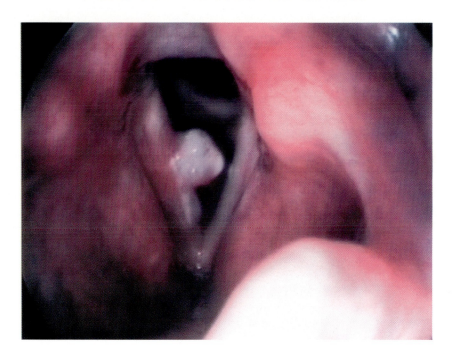

This 55-year-old engineer (a nonsmoker) has a squamous cell carcinoma-in-situ of the right true vocal fold. Co-factors, such as second-hand smoke, vocal abuse, and gastroesophageal reflux disease must be considered in the etiology. This patient underwent a 24-hour pH probe examination and demonstrated severe gastroesophageal reflux disease.

D. Invasive Carcinoma

Case 69: T1 larynx

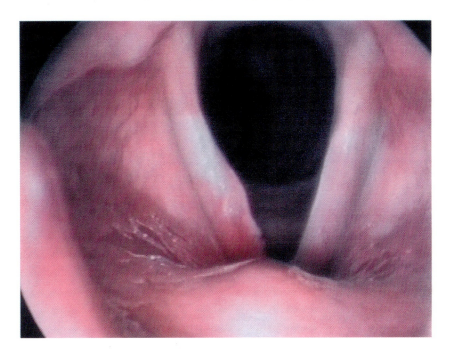

This 64-year-old executive with a 50 pack-year tobacco abuse history (he stopped smoking 10 years prior to his first visit to the Texas Voice Center) gave the chief complaint of persistent hoarseness for 7 months. Videostrobolaryngoscopy demonstrates a T1NoMo squamous cell carcinoma of the right true fold. The bulk, lack of mucosal wave, and discoloration of the right fold are apparent when compared to the more normal left fold.

Pathophysiology

The effect of the carcinoma within the right vocal fold is to dramatically increase the stiffness of the vocal fold reducing its ability to participate in vibrations. The increase in stiffness due to cancer typically results in either a reduction or the absence of any mucosal wave on the affected fold.

Case 70: T1 Squamous cell carcinoma of the pyriform sinus

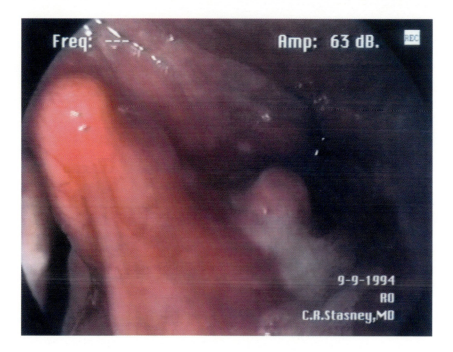

This case demonstrates another value of videostrobolaryngoscopy. This 71-year-old nonsmoker is a well-known Broadway actor who came to the Texas Voice Center complaining "I have no energy and my voice has not been dependable for the past 8 months." There is paradoxical vocal fold movement with diminished mucosal wave, but the significant finding is in the left pyriform sinus where a 5 mm exophytic lesion is seen. This proved to be a T1NoMo invasive squamous cell carcinoma—certainly the smallest one seen by the author and one of the few presenting without neck metastases.

Pathophysiology

The differences between the stiffness of the two vocal folds has resulted in vibrations that are at the same rate but appear to be out of phase with one another. The MDD demonstrates that there are irregularities primarily in the short-term and long-term cycle-to-cycle variations of the amplitude. The increased value of ATRI (Amplitude Tremor Related Index) indicates that there is a low frequency modulation of the amplitude. This modulation is due to the tremor that is readily apparent by viewing the supraglottic tissue during the stroboscopy. Although not present in the video sample, there are times when the tremor component increases, resulting in an intermittent breakdown of the voicing, accounting for the increased value of DUV (Degree of Voiceless) seen on the MDD (Fig 70).

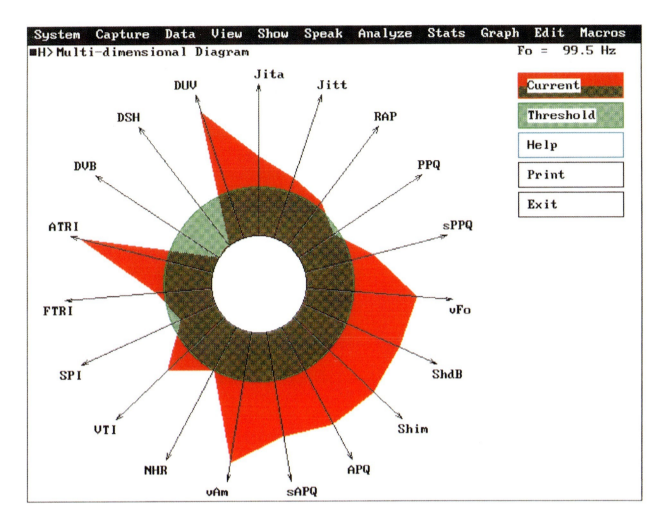

Fig 70

Case 71: T3 squamous cell carcinoma of the larynx

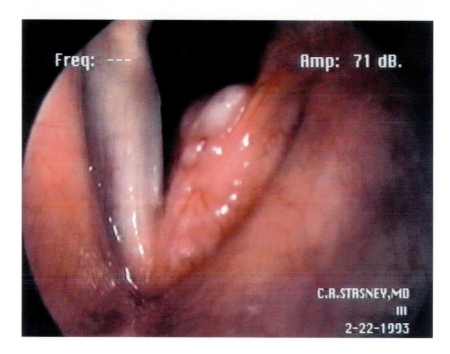

This patient is a 60-year-old housewife from Mexico City. She is a nonsmoker, but has been breathing the air in Mexico City all her life. She complained of a long history of heartburn and said that the physicians in Mexico had treated her for "gastritis and a diaphragmatic hernia."

Before presenting to the Texas Voice Center, she had undergone two microlaryngoscopies in Mexico, neither of which demonstrated a malignancy. On videostroboscopy, the swollen, firm, immobile right fold is apparent, which on biopsy proved to be a T3NoMo squamous cell carcinoma.

Pathophysiology

This case shows how the invasion of carcinoma dramatically increases the stiffness component of the vocal folds eliminating them from participating in vocal fold vibrations.

Case 72: T4 squamous cell carcinoma of the pyriform sinus

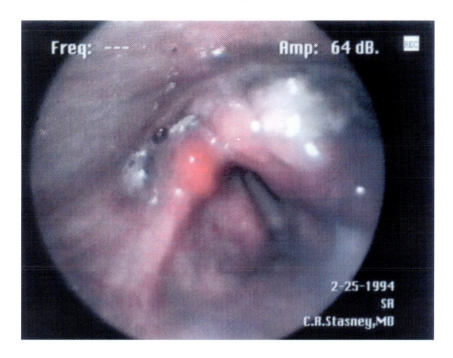

This 70-year-old executive with a 60 pack-year tobacco abuse history (he quit 25 years prior to his first visit) presented to the Texas Voice Center with complaints of dysphagia, odynophagia, left otalgia, and weight loss over the previous 6 months. The patient also suffered from arteriosclerotic cardiovascular disease and diabetes. The esophagoscopy and laryngoscopy with biopsies revealed a T4NoMo squamous cell carcinoma of the left pyriform extending into the endolarynx and upper esophagus.

Case 73: Verrucous carcinoma

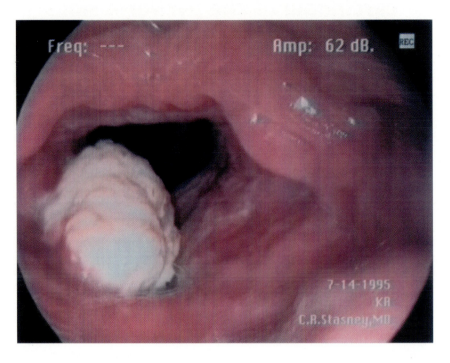

This is the case of a 62-year-old Saudi Arabian executive with a 90 pack-year history of tobacco abuse. A microlaryngoscopy was performed 11 years prior to his first visit to the Texas Voice Center which was consistent with verrucous carcinoma of the right false fold. The patient had been followed since that time without evidence of recurrence until this visit at which time the large verrucoid lesion visible on the right anterior false fold was noted. A repeat microlaryngoscopy with biopsy and laser debulking of the lesion was performed. The majority of the pathological specimen was consistent with verrucous carcinoma; however, a small focus of invasive squamous cell carcinoma was found and the patient had post-operative radiotherapy.

Verrucous carcinoma is a well-differentiated variant of squamous cell carcinoma.[29] The diagnosis is made by careful histopathology combined with clinical information. The human papilloma virus (especially HPV-16 and HPV-18) has been associated with the lesion.[30] For years, the hallmark of treatment was surgery as these lesions were thought to be refractory to irradiation and might even undergo anaplastic transformation. Recently, however, reports show that radiotherapy may have a place in the therapeutic armamentarium.[31]

IX. NEUROLOGIC DISORDERS

A. Nerve Paresis and Paralysis

Case 74: Bilateral superior laryngeal nerve paralyses

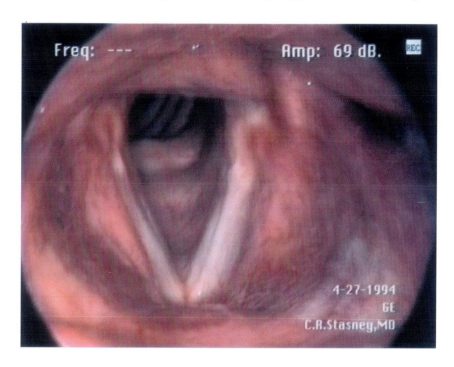

This 78-year-old patient complained of progressive hoarseness. The dysphonia began 4 weeks following a course of chemotherapy for lymphoma. On videostroboscopy, normal mobility of the arytenoids with adequate closure of the vocal processes is noted. There is, however, significant flaccidity of the vocal folds consistent with bilateral cricothyroid dysfunction (and therefore, bilateral superior laryngeal nerve paralyses).

Isolated superior laryngeal nerve (SLN) paralysis is very difficult to diagnose. Some of the ideas of rotation and elevation of the vocal folds after SLN paralysis have been questioned by recent studies by Koufman et al. in which he demonstrated that the cricothyroid muscle does not predictably influence the position of the vocal fold in unilateral paralysis.[32] In bilateral cases, even though this patient did not have an EMG to prove the diagnosis, the vocal folds are limp and the overall functional appearance of the larynx is consistent with bilateral superior laryngeal nerve paralyses with the resultant loss of cricothyroid function.

Pathophysiology

Consistent with the diagnosis of bilateral SLN paralysis, the patient's speech pattern is monotone in nature with a complete inability to modify the pitch. When viewing the stroboscopy, it is apparent that the inability to increase the longitudinal tension by increasing the length of the vocal folds due to the SLN paralysis is compensated by excessive amounts of medial-lateral compression. The medial-lateral compression becomes so extensive at times that the ventricular or false folds begin to participate in the vibrations, resulting in the diplophonia that is characteristic of the patient's speech. The MDD (Fig 74) demonstrates extreme abnormalities in nearly all of the parameters. There is very little regularity in the vocal fold vibrations both in the short- and long-term analyses. The inability to approximate the central portion of the folds produces excessive noise in the signal resulting in higher values of VTI (Voice Turbulence Index) and NHR (Noise to Harmonic Ratio).

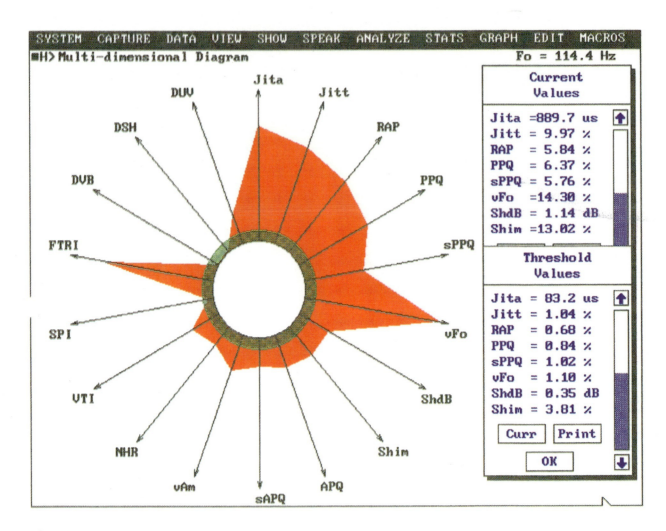

Fig 74

Case 75: Unilateral recurrent laryngeal nerve paralysis

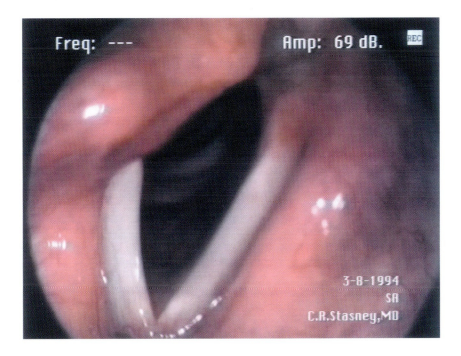

This 47-year-old female presented with hoarseness since awakening from knee surgery 4 days previous. Until the surgical procedure, her voice was reported as normal. Reports of paralyzed recurrent laryngeal nerve(s) following endotracheal intubation (but without surgery near the nerves, e.g., thyroidectomy, thoracic aneurysm, etc.) have been reported, but their exact etiology is unknown. Perhaps they occur secondary to pressure on the nerve by an endotracheal tube cuff. Many of these paralyses are temporary and resolve with time.

Pathophysiology

Perceptually this patient's voice is characterized by extreme breathiness with intermittent voicing occurring primarily at the initiation of phonation. When viewing the stroboscopy, the immobility of the right vocal fold is readily apparent. The approximation of the vocal folds occurs only when the mobile left vocal fold is adducted to the extent that it crosses the midline. To achieve this hyperadduction, medial compression is increased, as can be seen by the bulging of the ventricular fold. The quality of the voice achieved by patients with recurrent laryngeal nerve (RLN) paralysis is dependent primarily on the ability of the mobile fold to approximate with the immobile fold. Some patients with RLN damage are able to achieve relatively good voicing. This is particularly the case when the immobile fold lies fairly close to the midline and maintains a relatively straight edge to the vibrating margin.

Case 76: Bilateral recurrent laryngeal nerve paralyses

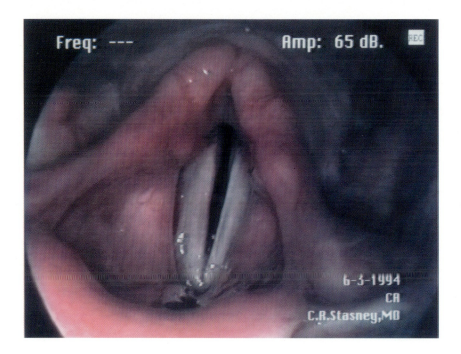

This 41-year-old female nurse underwent a bilateral thyroidectomy 7 months before presenting to the Texas Voice Center. She stated that she was immediately hoarse upon awakening from surgery and her voice had not improved in the interval prior to being seen. Furthermore, she had significant stridor on even mild exertion.

Pathophysiology

The RLNs supply the posterior cricoarytenoid, lateral cricoarytenoid, thyroarytenoid, and interarytenoid muscles. During the inspiratory process, the posterior cricoarytenoid muscles are responsible for abducting the folds to establish an increased glottal width for inspiration. During voicing, the lateral cricoarytenoid, thyroarytenoid, and interarytenoid muscles are responsible for adducting the vocal folds to place the vocal folds in the appropriate configuration to produce vocal fold vibrations. This patient clearly demonstrates the trade-off that occurs between the ability to produce voicing and the ability to open the glottis to achieve adequate inspiration. If the vocal folds are fixed relatively close to the midline, adequate voicing is possible; but the patient has difficulty abducting the vocal folds for inspiration. If, on the other hand, the vocal folds are fixed in a wider position, inspiration is easily achieved; but the patient may not be able to obtain any voicing. This patient's vocal folds at rest are relatively close to the midline, and she maintains a slight ability to adduct the folds which explains her ability to produce phonation. Her inability to abduct the vocal folds during inspiration results in the blockage of the airstream producing the vocal fold vibrations that are characteristic of laryngeal stridor. The laryngeal stridor increases when increased inspiratory effort is required during physical exertion.

B. Spasmodic Dysphonia

Case 77: Adductor spasmodic dysphonia

This 44-year-old housewife noted progressive difficulty speaking beginning 18 months before her first visit to the Texas Voice Center. This case demonstrates the typical strangled voice of the disorder. On videostroboscopic examination, the fine tremor and episodic hyperadduction of the vocal folds are apparent.

Spasmodic dysphonia is a variant of focal dystonia involving involuntary spastic adduction of the vocal folds. A more common and well-known variant of focal dystonia is that of essential blepharospasm. The etiology is unknown at this time, but it is felt to have a central nervous system origin with peripheral manifestations. The spastic contractions can involve any combination of laryngeal muscles and can include such extra-laryngeal muscles as the tongue, hypopharyngeal musculature, and so on. There are two main variants of spasmodic dysphonia (or spasmodic dystonia), adductor and abductor. The adductor variety is demonstrated in case 77 and the abductor in case 78. These disorders are more easily and clearly differentiated with the ear than with the eye; however, the salient points of differentiation are typified in these videostroboscopic examples. Rodriquez and Ford used EMG to distinguish between the adductor and abductor variety; but in the experience of the Texas Voice Center the diagnosis is usually fairly clear unless the patient has a mixed variety.[33] Work by Van Pelt et al. demonstrates that the muscle activation patterns of spasmodic dysphonia are relatively normal in the interval between spasms; however, "symptoms occur when spasmodic bursts intrude on all otherwise normal pattern."[34]

There is almost always a component of hyperfunction in each case of spasmodic dysphonia, and this must be taken into consideration vis-à-vis therapy.

Pathophysiology

The most common perceptual descriptors used for patients with adductor spasmodic dysphonia are a strained, strangled voice with intermittent voice breaks. It is our belief that the characteristic speech pattern of spasmodic dysphonia is due to both a neurological and functional component. The neurological component produces the characteristic tremor seen in this patient and produces an excessive amount of muscle activity. The functional component, referred to simply as hyperfunction, is made up of the changes in the motor control patterns that the patient uses to compensate for the neurological component. The functional component also includes an increased amount of muscle activity in the laryngeal muscles and the surrounding muscles. This is most likely due to the natural tendency for muscle tension to spread, since overactivity of a particular motor neuron pool rarely remains confined to an isolated muscle group. When viewing the stroboscopy, two factors characteristic of adductor spasmodic dysphonia should be noted. First is the presence of tremor that often involves both the vocal folds and the supraglottic muscles. In some patients, the tremor can be noted in the pharyngeal walls and soft palate. The excessive medial-lateral compression of the vocal folds is also characteristic of this disorder. The bulging of the ventricular or false folds inward is characteristic of the medial-lateral compression. At times the compression is so extensive that the glottis is completely closed off, resulting in the voice breaks and strangled sound that are so characteristic of adductor spasmodic dysphonia. Acceptance of the co-existence of the neurological and functional components most likely accounts for the therapeutic success that occurs when medical treatment is combined with functional voice treatment and perhaps accounts for the lack of success when only one component is treated in isolation.

Case 78: Abductor spasmodic dysphonia

This 57-year-old physician's spouse noted progressive difficulty speaking beginning 15 years before her first visit to the Texas Voice Center. Listen to the patient's voice and notice that, rather than a strangled sound, one hears a breathier voice and that prolonged vowel sounds tend to break off. Her voice is somewhat akin to that of a person who has been weeping.

The abductor variety is primarily due to episodic spasms in the posterior cricoarytenoid muscle which prevent prolonged voicing by abducting the vocal folds. Support for this hypothesis is gleaned not only from EMG work,[35] but also from the results of therapy which demonstrate temporary relief of symptoms when botulinum toxin is injected into the posterior cricoarytenoid muscle for the abductor variety.[36]

Pathophysiology

Perceptually this patient's speech is characterized by regular bursts of extreme breathiness. During these periods the voicing frequently ceases due to the contraction of the posterior cricoarytenoid muscles. The significant amount of air escaping during these periods requires greater respiratory effort on the part of the patient or more frequent breaths. The incoordination that the patient has on repetitive tasks that require alternating abduction and adduction (e.g., "he-he-he") is readily apparent when viewing the stroboscopy. At times excessive medial-lateral compression is present, most likely a compensatory behavior devised to prevent the vocal folds from inadvertently abducting. The abductor type is the most uncommon type of spasmodic dysphonia, occurring in 5 to 10% of spasmodic dysphonia patients.

C. Miscellaneous Neurological Disorders

Case 79: Paradoxical vocal fold dysfunction

This 42-year-old legal secretary noticed the acute onset of aphonia 7 days after getting a flu shot and 6 weeks before presenting to the Texas Voice Center. In addition, the act of trying to phonate caused her to be dyspneic. An initial diagnosis of asthma was made but therapy proved ineffective. Note the adduction of the folds on inspiration and the abduction on expiration—just the opposite of normal physiology.

Paradoxical vocal fold dysfunction is a rare disorder involving adduction of the folds during inspiration and abduction during expiration. The diagnosis is readily apparent from videostroboscopic examination of this patient. It is very important to make the proper diagnosis because this disorder can lead to fatalities.[37] Not infrequently (as in case 79), the initial diagnosis is asthma, but most often, the anti-asthma therapy is not effective.[38]

Pathophysiology

This patient, like most patients with paradoxical vocal fold dysfunction, performs better when breathing through the nose than when breathing through the mouth. When breathing through the nose, there is an increase in the resistance to the airstream resulting in increased negative air pressure within the lungs. The patient's greater success in achieving abduction using nasal breathing may be due to the powerful reflexive link between the pulmonary receptors and the posterior cricoarytenoid muscles used during inspiration. The development of therapeutic techniques for treating paradoxical vocal fold dysfunction has only recently occurred. It is our belief that the use of increased resistance to flow, either by using nasal breathing or inspiring through pursed lips, may enhance the ability to retrain the laryngeal muscles.

X. HORMONAL IMBALANCES

Case 80: Male (hypogonadism)

This 28-year-old CPA presented to the Texas Voice Center with the chief complaint "I want to lower my speaking voice." He stated that the pitch of his speaking voice did not lower significantly after puberty.

There is a wide variant of "normal," and this case merely represents one end of the normal spectrum. The relatively short, thin folds are more typical of a female appearance than a male and the patient's higher fundamental frequency demonstrates this fact. However, the patient's testosterone level and other male characteristics (hair distribution, gonad development, etc.) were within normal limits.

Case 81: Female with androgen effect

This 25-year-old female country and western singer presented with the chief complaint: "I have a lot of thickness in my throat, hoarseness and I haven't been able to perform (sing) at all for the past 20 months." The patient had been diagnosed with endometriosis in another state and given frequent, large doses of testosterone over a 2-year span in an attempt to ameliorate the symptoms of the gynecologic disease.

Unfortunately, this patient suffered from endometriosis and was treated with (what many might call excessive) repeated injections of testosterone. She developed several male traits, including a lowered fundamental frequency (probably secondary to thickened vocal folds), and a male pattern of hair distribution (including chest and facial hair).

XI. PEDIATRIC LARYNGEAL DISORDERS

As a postscript for this atlas, we elected to include a selection of pediatric cases, not only to demonstrate some of the more common diagnoses of childhood, but also to demonstrate that the videostroboscopic examination techniques apply to our young patients as well.

A. Nodules

Case 82: Nodules

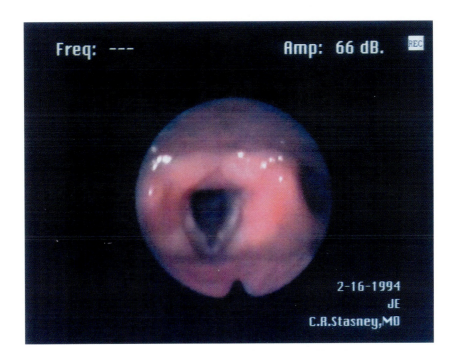

This 4-year-old female was reported by her mother to have had a deep, raspy voice since birth.

The typical appearance of callous-type lesions at the juncture of the anterior and middle thirds of the vocal folds is easily seen. These lesions are relatively common in young children with effusive personalities who make their presence known. Hearing loss must be excluded as this is an etiologic factor in development of nodules (please see case 84).

Case 83: Nodules

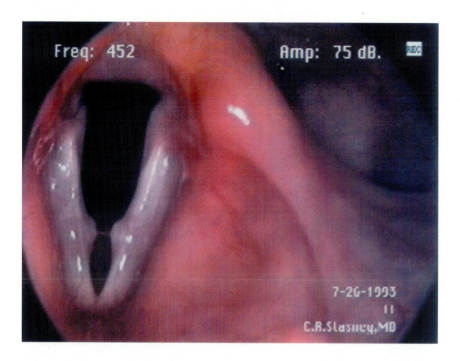

This 8-year-old female musical theater actress became severely hoarse during performances of the Annie role. The large, hyperkeratotic nodules at the juncture of the anterior and middle thirds of both vocal folds are easily seen.

The "Annie role" is very difficult, if not impossible, for children to perform without injury to their larynges. The tessitura and belting requirements are extreme, and many children have suffered vocal damage by performing roles such as this one. "Stage parents," much like "tennis parents," must be admonished not to push their children into demanding roles and vocal exercises which may cause injury.

Case 84: Nodules

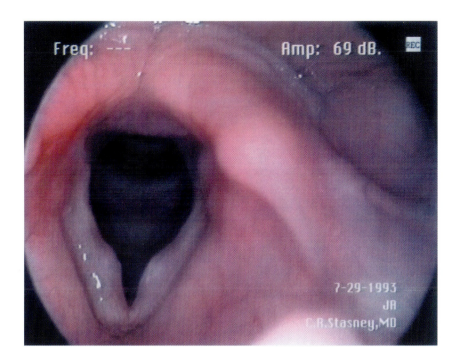

This 7-year-old male suffered from recurrent bouts of serous otitis media for which he underwent multiple myringotomies with tube insertions. Scarred tympanic membranes with a 20 decibel hearing loss were noted on audiometric evaluation, and the mother stated that the child had a hearing loss more often than not in spite of the repeated tube insertions. The more sessile appearance of this young patient's nodules (compared with those in case 83) demonstrate the variety of appearances of vocal nodules.

This child's primary etiologic cause for nodules was his hearing loss caused by multiple recurrent bouts of otitis and chronic serous otitis media. Before beginning speech therapy, the child's hearing should be assessed, and any abnormalities should be corrected either by surgery or by amplification.

B. Polyps

Case 85: Polyp

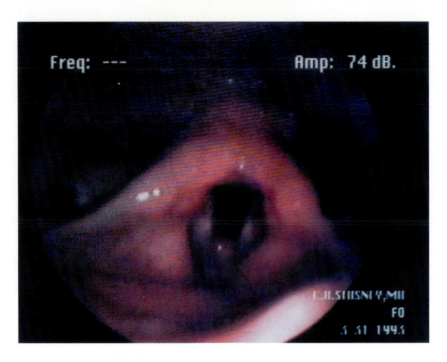

This 5-year-old female had a significant voice change in the 3 months prior to her first visit to the Texas Voice Center. Otolaryngologists in another country were unable to find the cause of the change in her voice. A typical angiomatous polyp is noted arising from the anterior commissure which deflects superiorly on forced phonation. This lesion typifies the reason to perform a flexible fiberoptic examination in order to make a definitive diagnosis and not to assume that all hoarseness in children is due to vocal nodules.

Patience and persistence are the hallmarks in examination of children, and one notes the distinct advantage of videostroboscopy in this case when a one second glimpse of the lesion can be expanded via a slow-motion effect.

C. Cysts

Case 86: Intracordal cyst

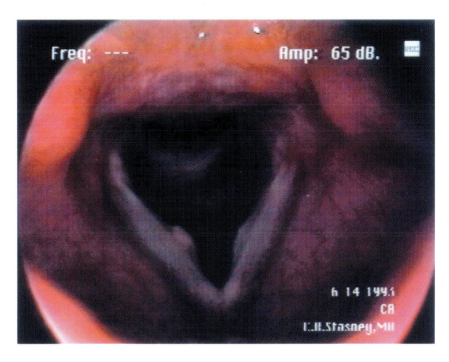

This 10-year-old male presented with a 6-month history of hoarseness. The lesion seen on videostroboscopy is consistent with the diagnosis of a right intracordal cyst with left nodule at the contact point. In this particular case, prolonged speech therapy, assuming that this patient had vocal nodules, would again be met with frustration. This is not to say that there is not an important place for speech therapy in the rehabilitation of these patients once a diagnosis is made and possible surgical intervention carried out. However, as a sole means of therapy, it has a small incidence of success for like lesions. Remember that saccular cysts can occur in infants and be a source of airway compromise[39] and that subglottic cysts can occur in children after long-term intubation.[40]

Epilogue

We hope this treatise has helped you in evaluations of laryngeal pathology. At the Texas Voice Center, we firmly believe in the team approach to the complete evaluation and treatment of laryngeal disorders, whether they are functional or organic. Please use this as a reference and do not hesitate to contact any of the authors by letter or telephone ([713] 796-2001) if you have questions.

We have attempted to demonstrate the videostroboscopic appearance of many lesions and have emphasized the diagnosis, not the treatment. Many excellent treatment texts have been published, and the authors refer you to some of them for additional information:

1. *Phonosurgery for Benign Vocal Fold Lesions*, Marc Bouchayer, M.D., Guy Cornut, M.D., The Three Ears Company Limited, London, 1994.
2. *Microlaryngoscopy and Endolaryngeal Microsurgery*, Oskar Kleinsasser, M.D., Hanley and Belfus, Inc., Philadelphia, 1990.
3. *Voice Surgery*, Wilbur James Gould, M.D., Robert Thayer Sataloff, M.D., D.M.A., Joseph Richard Spiegel, M.D., Mosby, Philadelphia, 1993.
4. *Diagnosis and Treatment of Voice Disorders*, John S. Rubin, M.D., Robert Thayer Sataloff, M.D., D.M.A., Gwen S. Korovin, M.D., Wilbur James Gould, M.D., Igaku-Shoin, New York, 1995.
5. *Phonosurgery*, Charles N. Ford, M.D., Diane M. Bless, Ph.D., Raven Press, New York, 1991.
6. *Phonosurgery*, Nobuhiko Isshiki, M.D., Springer-Velag, Tokyo, 1989.

Many thanks from all of us at the Texas Voice Center and Van Lawrence Voice Institute.

References

1. Kleinsasser O. *Microlaryngoscopy and Endolaryngeal Microsurgery*. Philadelphia: Hanley and Belfus Inc; 1991.
2. Suhonen PO et al. Saccular cyst of the larynx in infants. *Int J Ped Otol*. 1984;8:73–78.
3. Newman BH et al. Laryngeal cysts in adults: a clinicopathologic study of 20 cases. *Am J Clin Pathol*. 1984;81:715–720.
4. Som PM et al. Thyroglossal duct cysts that mimic laryngeal masses. *Laryngoscope*. 1987;97:742–745.
5. Toriumi DM et al. Acquired subglottic cysts in premature infants. *Int J Ped Otol*. 1987;14:151–160.
6. Oliveira CA et al. Oncocytic lesions of the larynx. *Laryngoscope*. 1977; 87:1718-1725.
7. Maier W et al. Pathogenic and therapeutic aspects of contact granuloma. *Laryngorhinootologie*. 1994;73:488–491.
8. Miko TL. Peptic (contact ulcer) granuloma of the larynx. *J Clin Pathol*. 1989;42: 800–804.
9. Benjamin B et al. Giant Teflon granuloma of the larynx. *Head and Neck*. 1991;13:453–456.
10. Lebovics RS et al. The management of subglottic stenosis and other communication disorders, National Institutes of Health. *Laryngoscope*. 1992;102:1341–1345.
11. Jindal JR et al. Gastroesophageal reflux disease as a likely cause of "idiopathic" subglottic stenosis. *Ann Otol Rhinol Laryngol*. 1994;103:186–191.
12. Koufman JA. The otolaryngologic manifestations of gastroesophageal reflux disease (GERD): a clinical investigation of 225 patients using ambulatory 24-hour pH monitoring and an experimental investigation of the role of acid and pepsin in the development of laryngeal injury. *Laryngoscope*. 1991; 101(4 pt. 2 suppl. 53):1–78.
13. Copova M et al. Gastroesophageal reflux as the basis of recurrent and chronic respiratory diseases. *Cesk Pediatr*. 1991;46:142–145.
14. Contencin P et al. Nasopharyngeal pH monitoring in infants and children with chronic rhinopharyngitis. *Int J Pediat Otol*. 1991;22:249–256.
15. Lacy PD et al. Late congenital syphilis of the larynx and pharynx presenting at endotracheal intubation. *Laryngol and Otol*. 1994;108:688–689.
16. Espinoza CG et al. Laryngeal tuberculosis. *Laryngoscope*. 1981;91:110–113.
17. Titche LL. Causes of recurrent laryngeal nerve paralysis. *Arch Otol*. 1976;102:259–261.
18. Sataloff RT et al. Vocal fold hemorrhagic mass: functional implications. *ENT*. 1994; 74:114.
19. Bouchayer M et al. *Phonosurgery for Benign Vocal Fold Lesions*. London: The Three Ears Company Ltd; 1994:55.
20. Bouchayer M et al. *Phonosurgery for Benign Vocal Fold Lesions*. London: The Three Ears Company Ltd; 1994:61.
21. Stasney CR. Laryngeal webs: A new treatment for an old problem. *J Voice*. 1995;9:106–109.
22. Thompson JW et al. Epidermolysis bullosa dystrophica of the larynx and trachea. *Ann Otol*. 1980;89:428–429.
23. Glossop LP et al. Epidermolysis bullosa letalis in the larynx causing acute respiratory failure: A case presentation and review of the literature. *Int J Ped Otorhinolaryngology*. 1984;7:281–288.
24. Woo P et al. Diagnosis and treatment of persistent dysphonia after laryngeal surgery: A retrospective analysis of 62 patient. *Laryngoscope*. 1994;104:1084–1091.
25. Corbitt G et al. Human papillomavirus (HPV) genotypes associated with laryngeal papilloma. *J Clin Pathol*. 1988;41:284–288.
26. Siegel SE et al. Malignant transformation of tracheobronchial juvenile papillomatosis without prior radiotherapy. *Ann Otol Rhinol Laryngol*. 1979;88:192–197.

27. Benjamin B et al. Laryngoscopic diagnosis of laryngeal sarcoid. *Ann Otol Rhinol Laryngol.* 1995;104:529–531.
28. Galvan GL, Landis JN. Sarcoidosis of the larynx: preserving and restoring airway and professional voice. *J Voice.* 1993;7:81–94.
29. Longarela H et al. Verrucous carcinoma of the larynx. *Acta Otol.* 1995;46:49–52.
30. Fliss DM et al. Laryngeal verrucous carcinoma: a clinicopathologic study and detection of human papillomavirus using polymerase chain reaction. *Laryngoscope.* 1994; 104:146–152.
31. O'Sullivan B et al. Outcome following radiotherapy in verrucous carcinoma of the larynx. *Int J Radiat Oncol Biol Phys.* 1995;32: 611–617.
32. Koufman JA et al. The cricothyroid muscle does not influence vocal fold position in laryngeal paralysis. *Laryngoscope.* 1995;105: 368–372.
33. Rodriquez AA, Ford CN et al. Electromyographic assessment of spasmodic dysphonia patients prior to botulinum toxin injection. *Electromyogr Clin Neurophysiol.* 1994;34: 403–407.
34. Van Pelt F et al. Comparison of muscle activation patterns in adductor and abductor spasmodic dysphonia. *Ann Otol Rhinol and Laryngol.* 1994;103:192–200.
35. Watson BC et al. Laryngeal electromyographic activity in adductor and abductor spasmodic dysphonia. *Speech and Hear Res.* 1991;34:473–482.
36. Rontal M et al. A method for the treatment of abductor spasmodic dysphonia with botulinum toxin injections: a preliminary report. *Laryngoscope.* 1991;101:911–914.
37. Schafer H, von Wichert P. Functional obstruction of the upper airways as an expression of psychogenic vocal cord dysfunction. Fatal outcome of a functional disorder. *Med Klin.* 1993;88:548–552.
38. Irie M et al. A case of vocal cord dysfunction diagnosed as bronchial asthma, that was improved by psychosomatic therapy. *Nippon Kyobu Shikkan Gakkai Zasshi:* 1992;30:930–934.
39. Suhonen H et al. Saccular cyst of the larynx in infants. *Int J Ped Otol.* 1984;8:73–78.
40. Toriumi DM et al. Acquired subglottic cysts in premature infants. *Int J Ped Otol.* 1987;14:151–160.